MAKING SENSE
of ACUTE
MEDICINE

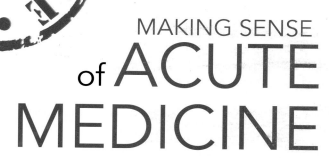

MAKING SENSE
of ACUTE
MEDICINE

A GUIDE TO
DIAGNOSIS

Paul F Jenkins
MA MB BChir FRCP FRCPE FRACP
Winthrop Professor of Medicine,
Faculty of Medicine, Dentistry and Health
Sciences, University of Western Australia,
Royal Perth Hospital and Joondalup Health
Campus, Perth, Australia

Paula H Johnson
MBChB DM FRCP
Associate Professor of Medicine, University
of Western Australia and Consultant General
and Respiratory Physician, Fremantle
Hospital, Fremantle, Australia

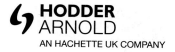

HODDER
ARNOLD
AN HACHETTE UK COMPANY

First published in Great Britain in 2010 by
Hodder Arnold, an imprint of Hodder Education, an Hachette UK company,
338 Euston Road, London NW1 3BH

http://www.hodderarnold.com

Whilst the advice and information in this book are believed to be true and accurate
at the date of going to press, neither the authors nor the publisher can accept any
legal responsibility or liability for any errors or omissions that may be made. In
particular (but without limiting the generality of the preceding disclaimer) every
effort has been made to check drug dosages; however it is still possible that errors
have been missed. Furthermore, dosage schedules are constantly being revised and
new side-effects recognized. For these reasons the reader is strongly urged to
consult the drug companies' printed instructions before administering any of the
drugs recommended in this book.

British Library Cataloguing in Publication Data
A catalogue record for this book is available from the British Library

Library of Congress Cataloging-in-Publication Data
A catalog record for this book is available from the Library of Congress

ISBN-13 978-0-340-98425-3

1 2 3 4 5 6 7 8 9 10

Commissioning Editor:	Joanna Koster
Project Editor:	Sarah Penny and Jane Tod
Production Controller:	Kate Harris
Cover Design:	Amina Dudhia
Indexer:	Lisa Footitt

Typeset in 11.5/13 pt ChaparralMM by MPS Limited, A Macmillan Company,
Chennai, India

Printed and bound in India

What do you think about this book? Or any other Hodder Arnold title?
Please visit our website: www.hodderarnold.com

Contents

Preface

This book is a guide to decision-making in Acute Medicine – a practical approach to the differential diagnosis of patients presenting as emergencies on the 'medical intake'.

Remarkable technological advances have been made in diagnostic medicine during the last 30 years. Examples include the development of magnetic resonance imaging (MRI), positron emission tomography (PET), spiral computerized tomography (CT), cardiac troponins, biochemical tumour markers, and numerous endoscopic and interventional radiological procedures. However, the appropriate use and interpretation of these tests remains dependent on the clinical skills, decision-making and analytical capabilities of the doctors who request them. Clever tests are no substitute for sound clinical skills and may actually mislead practitioners who lack the ability to use them appropriately. To use a crude analogy, a bad driver will drive a car badly regardless of whether it is a battered old Ford or a brand new Ferrari – and neither will get him to his destination if he makes an error of judgement leading to an accident on the way.

Competent physicians have many skills that underpin their practice of medicine and fundamental to these is the ability to take an accurate, comprehensive history (quickly) and perform a competent and directed physical examination. This results in an informed differential diagnosis which, in turn, dictates the requesting of focused diagnostic tests in order to narrow the differential diagnosis and guide the clinical management plan. The reader might consider that this is blindingly obvious;

but it is our experience that many medical students and junior doctors (and some more senior ones too) display poor clinical reasoning and decision-making skills and this results in their employing a 'scatter-gun' approach to diagnosis, suggesting or requesting multiple tests in the hope that the diagnosis will 'turn up' as a result. That is not good medicine. It exposes patients to unnecessary procedures and may uncover minor, irrelevant investigative abnormalities, which can result in additional unnecessary tests and may obscure the primary problem. The diagnostic art starts with excellent clinical skills.

Some new diagnostic techniques entail significant potential risk to patients. The obvious example is the risk posed by exposure to medical radiation as a result of the huge increase in radiological imaging that has occurred in recent years. Medical radiation is now the principal source of radiation exposure in the populations of developed countries. Given the wealth of increasingly complex technology now available to doctors, and the accompanying potential risks to patients, we believe that good reasoning and decision-making skills have never been more important in clinical medicine.

This book focuses on clinical decision-making as it applies to some major common presentations in acute medicine. Each chapter aims to analyse a medical presentation in a systematic way, and the reader is encouraged to apply logical thought at various stages particularly with regard to investigation and management.

This book is not intended to be a complete reference text for Acute Medicine. In particular, management is covered in outline only and not in detail as many other texts address management of acute medical problems. The topics covered relate to major common presentations to emergency medical services and not to specific diagnoses or physiological parameters (such as 'hypotension'). After all, patients do not attend emergency departments stating their diagnosis or complaining that they are hypotensive. To get the most out of this book it will be necessary to have a degree of background knowledge of common medical conditions. Our intention is to aid the clinical reasoning skills of medical students and trainee doctors as they learn to make the transition from clerking the patient to rationalizing differential diagnosis, requesting sensible and focused investigations, and formulating appropriate management plans.

Acknowledgements

The authors wish to thank Dr Peter Kendall and Dr Lena Thin for help in finding x-ray images for reproduction here.

List of abbreviations

α_1-AT	Alpha-1 antitrypsin
ACS	Acute coronary syndrome
ALP	Alkaline phosphatase
ALT	Alanine transaminase
ANA	Antinuclear antibody
ANCA	Antinuclear cytoplasmic antibody
AP	Anteroposterior
ARVD	Arrhythmogenic right ventricular dysplasia
ASD	Atrioseptal defect
AST	Aspartate transaminase
AVRT	Atrioventricular re-entrant tachycardia
BCT	Broad-complex tachycardia
BNP	Brain natriuretic peptide
BPPV	Benign paroxysmal positional vertigo
CBD	Common bile duct
CCF	Congestive cardiac failure
CK	Creatine phosphokinase
CMV	Cytomegalovirus
COPD	Chronic obstructive pulmonary disease
CRP	C-reactive protein
CSF	Cerebrospinal fluid
CT	Computerized tomography
CTEPH	Chronic thromboembolic pulmonary hypertension
CTPA	CT pulmonary angiogram
CXR	Chest x-ray
DIC	Disseminated intravascular coagulation
DKA	Diabetic ketoacidosis

DVT	Deep vein thrombosis
EBV	Epstein–Barr virus
ECG	Electrocardiograph
ECHO	Echocardiogram
EEG	Electroencephalography
EMG	Electromyography
ENA	Extractable nuclear antigen
ERCP	Endoscopic retrograde cholangiopancreatography
ESR	Erythrocyte sedimentation rate
FBC	Full blood count
GBS	Guillain–Barré syndrome
GCS	Glasgow Coma Scale
GGT	Gamma glutamyl transferase
GI	Gastrointestinal
GORD	Gastro-oesophageal reflux disease
GP	General practitioner
GTN	Glyceryl trinitrate
HCG	Human chorionic gonadotrophin
HCV	Hepatitis C virus
HFE gene	Haemochromatosis gene
HIV	Human immunodeficiency virus
HLA	Human leucocyte antigen
HPOA	Hypertrophic obstructive osteoarthropathy
HRCT	High-resolution computerized tomography
HSV	Herpes simplex virus
HVS	Hyperventilation syndrome
IBD	Inflammatory bowel disease
IgE	Immunoglobulin E
INR	International normalized ratio
IV	Intravenous
JVP	Jugular venous pressure
LDH	Lactate dehydrogenase
LMN	Lower motor neurone
LP	Lumbar puncture
LSD	Lysergic acid diethylamide
LVF	Left ventricular failure
MAP	Mean arterial pressure

MCH	Mean cell haemoglobin
MCV	Mean cell volume
MI	Myocardial infarction
mmHg	millimetres of mercury
MRCP	Magnetic resonance cholangiopancreatography
MRI	Magnetic resonance imaging
MSU	Mid-stream urine
NSAID	Non-steroidal anti-inflammatory drug
PA	Postero-anterior
PBC	Primary biliary cirrhosis
PCR	Protein creatinine ratio
PE	Pulmonary embolism
PET	Positron emission tomography
PHT	Pulmonary hypertension
PT	Prothrombin time
PUO	Pyrexia of unknown origin
RNP	Ribonucleoprotein
SAH	Subarachnoid haemorrhage
SDH	Subdural haemorrhage
SLE	Systemic lupus erythematosus
SSRI	Selective serotonin-reuptake inhibitor
SVT	Supraventricular tachycardia
TB	Tuberculosis
UMN	Upper motor neurone
V/Q	Ventilation/perfusion
VT	Ventricular tachycardia
VTE	Venous thromboembolism

To Glynis, David and Peter Jenkins – for many reasons.

Paul Jenkins

To Kate, Zoe and Zac for everything.

Paula Johnson

1 The shocked patient

● Introduction

Shock can be defined practically as *any clinical situation that results in inadequate tissue perfusion*. When this happens, tissue oxygen delivery is impaired and a number of metabolic consequences accrue as a result of increasing anaerobic metabolism. If this state is uncorrected, it will result in progressive organ dysfunction, multi-organ damage and, ultimately, death.

In the early stages of shock a patient may be relatively asymptomatic, as compensatory mechanisms – including sympathetically driven tachycardia and vasoconstriction – attempt to maintain a near normal blood pressure. As the degree of shock worsens, compensatory mechanisms eventually fail, blood pressure falls, and organ hypoperfusion results. At this stage, the patient will be symptomatic and manifest haemodynamic abnormalities with cool, clammy peripheries and a prolonged capillary refill time. Compromised end-organ perfusion of brain and kidney are evidenced, respectively, by restlessness and agitation and diminished urine output.

The mortality rate for shock from many causes still exceeds 50 per cent and its successful treatment demands prompt

● Classification of shock states

Hypovolaemic (oligaemic) shock

This group comprises any clinical state that results in reduced circulatory volume:

- Haemorrhage is commonly responsible. This may be obviously due to trauma or overt gastrointestinal bleeding, or covert as in occult gastrointestinal blood loss or retroperitoneal haemorrhage.
- Gastrointestinal fluid loss from diarrhoea, vomiting or both.
- Pathological salt and/or free water loss from the kidney as seen in primary renal disease (e.g. obstructive uropathy) or in endocrinological diseases such as Addison's disease or diabetes insipidus.
- Potentially severe fluid loss from skin pathology, including desquamative skin rashes and extensive burns.

Cardiogenic shock

Failure of the heart to maintain adequate systemic blood flow can have a number of causes:

- *Myocardial* (or 'pump') failure most commonly arises from the reduced systolic function that accompanies myocardial infarction. It can also complicate acute myocarditis or occur as an end result of cardiomyopathy.
- *Mechanical* failure can result from mitral valve rupture, rupture of a papillary muscle, or a traumatic ventricular septal defect. All of these acute mechanical events arise most commonly as complications of myocardial infarction.
- *Obstructive* (extracardiac) shock is seen in pericardial tamponade, massive pulmonary embolism or severe pulmonary hypertension.

Distributive shock

This is the term given to shock states where hypotension and tissue hypoperfusion result from an abnormal distribution of circulating fluids:

- *Septic* shock is the most commonly encountered example in this category. The development of shock in sepsis is complicated, but the first (distributive) element is generally an abnormal vasodilatation, which is a response to infection. This is then compounded by 'third space' fluid loss where circulating fluids leak into the extracellular space because of 'leaky capillaries', another fundamental pathophysiological response to sepsis.
- *Anaphylactic* shock is a severe allergic reaction that follows re-exposure to a foreign allergen (commonly a drug, food, foreign serum or venoms) to which a patient has been previously sensitized and produced IgE as a result. Re-exposure to the allergen releases mediators that result in vasodilatation, smooth muscle contraction, increased glandular secretion and increased capillary permeability. Shock can be the end-result of this process. Other clinical features include bronchospasm, upper airway obstruction, facial and tongue swelling, generalized or localized urticaria, angioneurotic oedema and abdominal pain.
- *Neurogenic* subtypes of shock are also best classified in the Distributive category. In this case, shock results from the loss of peripheral vasomotor tone that can complicate spinal cord injury, epidural or general anaesthesia and also follow administration of autonomic blocking agents. In each of these situations, peripheral blood pooling results in reduced tissue perfusion.

recognition and an awareness of the potential underlying differential diagnosis.

A classification of shock states is provided here, but it is important to realize that there is considerable overlap within the categories of shock. In sepsis, for example, the distributive element of shock arising from vasodilatation is compounded by hypovolaemia due to third-space fluid loss as well as myocardial dysfunction, which is a direct toxic effect of sepsis. Each of these three pathophysiological contributors to reduced tissue perfusion in septic shock can predominate at different stages of sepsis. Typically, vasodilatation is the initial dominant factor, followed by fluid shift as a result of 'leaky' capillaries. Finally, the clinical picture is complicated by the development of myocardial dysfunction as a toxic effect of generalized sepsis.

● History

Use the classification provided to guide a systematic history.

Hypovolaemic shock

- Is there a history of blood loss, excessive gastrointestinal loss from diarrhoea and/or vomiting, or burns?
- Inadequate fluid intake in a hot climate readily compounds other causes of hypovolaemia and is an important consideration in hot countries.
- Enquire also about excessive loss through the kidneys with symptoms of polyuria and/or nocturia.

Cardiogenic shock

- **Myocardial**. Is there a history suggestive of acute myocardial infarction, previous ischaemic heart disease or cardiomyopathy?
- **Mechanical**. As mentioned above, the majority of mechanical causes for cardiogenic shock complicate acute myocardial infarction.

- **Obstructive**. Enquire about any features in the history that might suggest major pulmonary embolism (PE). These include relevant risk factors for thromboembolic disease (covered in Chapter 3). Remember that typical pleuritic pain is often not a feature of large pulmonary emboli (see **Think** below).

Enquire also about features suggestive of pericardial disease. Pericarditic pain often has elements of typical 'crushing' ischaemic-sounding pain together with an exacerbation on deep inspiration that is indistinguishable from pleuritic chest pain. Recurrent pericarditis is most common in young men, and the pain is often associated with posture, being commonly (though not always) relieved on sitting up and leaning forward. Pericardial tamponade is unlikely to complicate acute pericarditis and is more commonly associated with malignancy, uraemia and sometimes bacterial infection.

THINK

What symptoms are common with large pulmonary emboli?

- Massive pulmonary embolism presents with sudden death or shock. Sub-massive PE is defined as absence of systemic hypotension but with evidence (usually echocardiographic) of right ventricular strain. Sudden breathlessness is more common than pleuritic chest pain in these settings.
- Remember that major pulmonary embolism can produce 'secondary' cardiac pain and even myocardial infarction by virtue of a sudden severe increase in afterload on the right ventricle and resulting increased demand for myocardial blood flow and oxygen. Cardiac pain with PE will be more likely if there is concomitant coronary artery disease.

Distributive shock

- **Septic**. Always question the possibility of sepsis in a shocked patient (see **Hazard** below). Is there any suggestion of recent infection or of a continuing source for sepsis? Your enquiry will need to be broad and include all potential sites for infection – respiratory, urinary tract, joints, bones, sinuses, and so on.
- **Anaphylactic**. Recent insect stings or bites are obvious avenues to explore if there is any suggestion of an anaphylactic reason for shock. In addition, ask about recent drug usage – and remember that an allergic response to drugs may not be immediate: it is not uncommon for penicillin allergy to manifest 7–10 days after commencing a course of the drug. Enquire about foodstuffs as well: common culprits for food allergy are nuts (which may be surprising components of various foods) and shellfish. A previous history of allergic responses will be helpful in making the diagnosis of anaphylactic shock.
- **Neurogenic**. The history is usually straightforward with evidence for recent trauma and spinal injury or a recent anaesthetic procedure.

HAZARD

Early diagnosis and management are crucial in securing a favourable outcome in septic shock.
- If shock is present, consider sepsis as the possible cause.
- Similarly, if a patient is septic, question whether they are shocked.

● Examination

There are some basic comments to be made first. A shocked patient presents clinically in one of two ways depending on whether the cardiac index is decreased (hypodynamic presentation) or increased (hyperdynamic presentation).

- **Hypodynamic presentation**. A low cardiac index is typical of both hypovolaemic and cardiogenic shock. The patient is poorly perfused with cool, clammy peripheries and a slow capillary refill time. Tachycardia is usually present as a result of an agonal chronotropic response. Tachypnoea is also common and is secondary to the metabolic acidosis caused by poor tissue perfusion. More specifically, reduced cerebral and renal perfusion result in mental confusion and oliguria, respectively.
- **Hyperdynamic presentation**. The cardiac index is usually high in cases of distributive shock and is classically so in sepsis. This hyperdynamic state means that hypotension is combined with warm peripheries, bounding peripheral pulses and a normal capillary refill time at least in the early stages of septic shock – all quite different from the findings in hypovolaemic and cardiogenic shock states.

Now consider the specific examination findings in different shock states.

Hypovolaemic shock
Hypotension (see **Hazard** below) and signs of poor tissue perfusion (cold, clammy peripheries and capillary refill time >2 s) are combined with:

- tachycardia
- tachypnoea
- confusion
- oliguria
- low central venous pressure (a jugular venous pressure that cannot be seen when the patient is lying flat is indicative of marked hypovolaemia).

HAZARD

A compensatory sympathetic response can maintain systemic blood pressure in the early stages of hypovolaemic shock. This is usually seen in young, previously fit individuals, whose blood pressure is maintained by progressive systemic vasoconstriction. Clinically, the clue to this adaptive response (which is usually blunted or absent in the elderly or infirm) is a rising diastolic blood pressure with a stable systolic pressure – in other words, a diminishing pulse pressure. It is important not to miss this physiological sign because compensatory mechanisms can fail suddenly with catastrophic consequences.

Cardiogenic shock

Hypotension and poor tissue perfusion are combined with:

- tachycardia
- tachypnoea
- confusion
- oliguria;

but a central venous pressure that is usually (though not always) elevated – that is, greater than +2 cm from the clavicle with the patient sitting at 45 degrees. This is the important distinction from hypovolaemic shock and, in addition, there may be:

- additional heart sounds or a summation gallop
- murmurs of aortic or mitral valve disease or of a ventricular septal defect
- a dyskinetic myocardium on palpation of the precordium
- evidence of heart failure
- a positive Kussmaul's sign (elevation of the JVP on inspiration) and/or pulsus paradoxus >12 mmHg, which are suggestive of cardiac tamponade.

Septic shock

Hypotension is combined with:

- warm, well-perfused peripheries and a normal capillary refill time (this is not true in late stages of septic shock)
- tachycardia
- tachypnoea
- confusion
- oliguria
- low central venous pressure.

In addition, look for specific evidence of infection. This will include:

- abnormal body temperature, which may be high or low
- evidence for a collection of infection: intra-abdominal, respiratory (including empyema), septic joints or bones, etc.
- central nervous system infection
- specific clinical features such as the petechial rash of meningococcal septicaemia (see **Hazard** below) or subcutaneous pustules of gonococcal or staphylococcal septicaemia.

THINK

What are the clinical features necessary to diagnose septic shock?
By definition, these are:
- a proven source of infection
- a mean arterial pressure (MAP) of <65 mmHg despite adequate fluid resuscitation, or the requirement of pharmacologic vasopressor agents to maintain a normal MAP (see Clinical tip below). (To put things in a clinical perspective, a MAP of <65 mmHg is diagnostic of a shock state.)

There must also be two or more of the following manifestations of systemic inflammation:
- tachypnoea
- tachycardia

- a white cell count that is either elevated or depressed
- a body temperature that is either high or low
- dysfunction of at least one end organ.

CLINICAL TIP

The mean arterial pressure is an important arbiter of tissue perfusion. It is easily calculated: measure the pulse pressure (systolic BP minus diastolic BP), divide this by 3, and add the result to the diastolic blood pressure. This calculation takes into account the differential times occupied by systole and diastole during the cardiac cycle in their contribution to mean arterial blood pressure.

HAZARD

The characteristic non-blanching, purpuric rash of meningococcal septicaemia clinches a specific infective diagnosis. However, the skin lesions may be *minimal at the outset* and may be confined to pressure areas such as the buttocks and the backs of the thighs, areas often overlooked during routine examination.

● Investigations

Basic blood tests are required in all cases of shock, and these include:

- full blood count, including a differential white cell count and platelet count
- clotting screen to look for evidence of disseminated intravascular coagulation

- serum creatinine, urea and electrolytes, including chloride (see **Hazard** below)
- liver function tests
- troponin level
- markers of inflammation, especially C-reactive protein.

HAZARD

Fluid resuscitation with large volumes of normal (0.9%) saline may result in hyperchloraemic metabolic acidosis. In this situation, crystalloid solutions containing less chloride (e.g. Hartmann's solution) should be used.

The possibility of *sepsis* must be considered in all shocked patients. Unless sepsis can be confidently excluded, blood cultures and other appropriate samples for culture are mandatory and should be taken, whenever practical, before antibiotics are commenced.

Additional tests are also indicated in most cases:

- arterial blood gases (see **Clinical tip** below)
- plasma lactate
- chest and abdominal radiographs
- electrocardiograph.

CLINICAL TIP

The interpretation of arterial blood gases should include analysis of acid–base balance and calculation of the alveolar–arterial oxygen difference using the modified alveolar gas equation. This is an easy calculation that provides information as to the efficiency of pulmonary gas exchange. The formula and its derivation are covered in all standard texts on respiratory physiology.

The following points should also be considered.

- Echocardiography is an invaluable tool in assessing left ventricular function or the presence of pericardial or valvular heart disease, as well as assisting in diagnosing pulmonary embolism by identifying right ventricular strain in major pulmonary embolism. It is important to recognize that transthoracic echocardiography may not exclude small vegetations of bacterial endocarditis, especially on the aortic valve – under these circumstances, transoesophageal echocardiography should be considered.
- Septic shock can result in either an elevation or a fall in the white cell count. It is important to note that the latter is associated with a particularly poor prognosis.
- An elevated C-reactive protein is a useful indicator of sepsis.
- Disseminated intravascular coagulation (DIC) is diagnosed by the combination of prolonged clotting, thrombocytopaenia and a reduced fibrinogen level. The presence of DIC has important management and prognostic implications.
- Plasma lactate is a marker of tissue hypoxia and is elevated in most cases of shock. The degree of elevation also correlates with the severity of the shock state. However, be aware that lactate levels may be artificially low during the early stages of fluid resuscitation because the accumulated tissue lactate is not being 'washed out' of the tissues in the presence of severe hypoperfusion. As the resuscitation proceeds, perfusion improves and there may be a rapid rise in lactate levels.
- CT pulmonary angiography (CTPA) is pivotal in confirming the diagnosis of pulmonary embolism and also helps to provide an anatomical assessment of the size of intrapulmonary arterial thrombus – the 'clot load'.
- CT scanning of the abdomen is indicated in suspected intra-abdominal pathology. Detection of a perforated viscus, infarcted bowel, abdominal aortic aneurysm or pancreatitis are all examples of its potential diagnostic utility.

2 The comatose patient

● Introduction

Consciousness is the normal (waking) state of awareness of self and the environment. *Coma* can therefore be defined as an absence of awareness even when one is externally stimulated. The presence of coma implies brain dysfunction that is either diffuse or multifocal.

THINK

What biological systems are necessary in order to render a person fully conscious?

Two basic neurological activities are needed.

- The first is 'alertness', a state of arousal that relies on a normally functioning ascending reticular activating system, situated in the mid-brain.
- The second is the ability to be aware of one's surroundings (and be able to respond to them appropriately). This is a function of the cerebral cortex. Put in another way, the combination of sensory information that informs an alert person regarding the details of his or her environment requires processing in the cerebral cortex for full 'awareness' to be present.

● Classification of coma

Structural pathologies
- *Vascular:*
  - Haemorrhage or infarction:
    - Cortical
    - Thalamic
    - Cerebellar
    - Brain-stem
  - Extradural haemorrhage
  - Subdural haemorrhage
  - Subarachnoid haemorrhage
  - Pituitary apoplexy
  - Cortical venous sinus thrombosis
  - Basilar artery aneurysm
- *Tumours:*
  - Primary
  - Secondary
- *Infection:*
  - Meningitis
  - Abscess
- *Head injury*
- *Demyelination:* particularly in brain-stem

Diffuse and/or metabolic brain dysfunction
- *Intrinsic diseases:*
  - Encephalitis
  - Concussion
  - Post-ictal states
- *Extrinsic disorders:*
  - Alcohol intoxication
  - Anoxia
  - Generalized ischaemia
  - Hypoglycaemia
  - Hepatic encephalopathy
  - Uraemia

- Hypothermia
- Hypothyroidism
- Drugs

Psychiatric 'coma'
- Conversion reactions: 'pseudo-coma'
- Depression
- Catatonic stupor

It follows that a reduced conscious level may have various causes.

- A lesion in the mid-brain can affect the centres for alertness, and/or pathology can affect higher cortical function. Neuro-anatomy explains that the lesion in the first instance may be quite small and is likely to be affecting other brain-stem centres, resulting in physical signs that may aid its localization.
- Diseases causing coma through disruption of the cortical function of awareness are likely to be far more extensive if structural in nature (e.g. a large intracerebral bleed), and may be accompanied by raised intracerebral pressure with resultant effects on the brain-stem as well as higher cortical function.
- Metabolic disturbances (e.g. hepatic encephalopathy) may reduce consciousness through a combined effect on brain-stem and cortical function.

These considerations introduce a clinical approach to the comatose patient that will aid speedy differential diagnosis.

In addition, there is an extreme priority in assessing comatose patients, namely to consider the possibility of *correctable causes* of coma. Correctable causes are predominantly metabolic or toxic in nature, and this chapter concludes with a systematic approach to identifying and coping with 'correctable coma'. Although this is not purely diagnostic information, we consider that the exclusion of correctable causes, their management and the potential pitfalls in management are sufficiently important to warrant inclusion here.

● History

It is vital to obtain as comprehensive a history as possible from relatives and other witnesses. In addition, search diligently for any previous medical history from hospital or GP records. The following historical features are critical.

Speed of onset

Sudden onset is typical of a vascular cause. Haemorrhage may be extradural, subdural, subarachnoid or intracerebral in site and extensive supratentorial bleeding into any of these sites is implicated if consciousness is depressed significantly. This also applies to intracerebral infarction when the area of cortex involved will be large and probably accompanied by surrounding oedema – producing a 'mass effect' with a resultant increase in intracranial pressure.

In the brain-stem, smaller vascular events (either haemorrhage or infarction) readily depress conscious level. The examination findings are crucial in clarifying the anatomical site of the lesion and in determining the likely prognosis.

A more gradual onset suggests alternative structural pathology, particularly a space-occupying lesion, and is more likely (although not exclusively so) if coma is metabolic or toxic in origin.

Accompanying headache

Sudden onset of severe headache is the cardinal symptom of subarachnoid haemorrhage (SAH). It is safe practice to assume that the cause of sudden severe headache is SAH until proved otherwise (see also Chapter 10).

Headache also accompanies primary intracerebral bleeding, when its onset may be sudden or more gradual in nature.

Headache can also occur in intracerebral infarction, but is less common.

Headache that has been present for longer periods, especially if associated with features suggestive of raised intracranial pressure (exacerbated by bending, coughing or straining at stool, for example), implies a space-occupying lesion.

Associated trauma

The history of trauma may be clear and temporally associated with the loss of consciousness; but be wary of earlier trauma that can be responsible for delayed intracranial bleeding – and this applies especially to subdural and extradural haemorrhage.

Additional symptoms

Ask for any clues that will identify the site and nature of the pathology. These will include preceding motor or sensory symptoms as well as brain-stem symptoms such as diplopia, dysarthria, dysphagia or ataxia.

Previous medical history

This is very important. Focus your questioning on a history of diabetes, epilepsy, previous episodes of loss of consciousness as well as anything suggestive of previous cardiovascular or cerebrovascular disease. Have there been any events that might be compatible with a malignant dysrhythmia? Is there a known history of excess alcohol consumption? Are there ongoing psychiatric problems? Is there a previous history of deliberate self-harm?

Family history

Is there a family history of premature vascular disease? Also, sudden death in the family raises the possibility of a malignant dysrhythmia or perhaps an inherited cardiomyopathy.

Social history

Question the possibility of clinical depression as well as drug or alcohol abuse. Specific questioning should include tablets,

medicines or empty pill (or other) bottles found in proximity
to the patient. Ambulance staff are helpful sources of this kind
of information.

● Examination

As always, a comprehensive general examination is necessary
as well as a detailed neurological assessment.

Depth of coma

Carefully assess the depth of coma using the Glasgow Coma
Scale (Table 2.1). Not only does this provide an objective
assessment of depth of coma on presentation, it also guides
the need for airway protection (a GCS of less than 9 generally
demands intubation) and provides a baseline as to whether the
patient is improving or deteriorating clinically.

General examination

● What is the respiratory rate and rhythm? The implications
  of this observation are discussed in detail under brain-stem
  signs.

Table 2.1 Glasgow Coma Scale

Eye opening Score 1–4	4 = spontaneous 3 = to verbal command 2 = to painful stimuli 1 = none
Verbal response Score 1–5	5 = oriented conversation 4 = disoriented conversation 3 = inappropriate words 2 = incomprehensible sounds 1 = none
Best motor response Score 1–6	6 = obeys verbal commands 5 = localizes painful stimuli 4 = flexion withdrawal from pain 3 = decorticate (flexion) response to pain 2 = decerebrate (extension) response to pain 1 = none

- Is there evidence of anaemia or jaundice?
- Are there stigmata of chronic liver disease?
- Does the patient smell of alcohol?
- Measure the core temperature of the patient.
- Is the patient malnourished, dishevelled or heavily tattooed? Are needle track marks evident or is there any other feature suggestive of drug abuse?
- Is there overt evidence of seizure activity? Be aware of the possibility of non-convulsive status epilepticus ('subtle status') (see Chapter 7) and look specifically for nystagmoid jerks of the eyes, myoclonic limb movements and akathisia.
- Are there any external injuries consistent with trauma? Examine the patient's head and scalp very carefully.

Cardiovascular, respiratory and abdominal systems

- Examine systematically for any organ-specific features that may provide clues to the cause of the coma (e.g. malignant dysrhythmia).
- Examine for any abnormalities that might be complications of the comatose state (e.g. aspiration pneumonia).

Neurological examination

Neurological examination has three fundamental aims: assess level of consciousness using the Glasgow Coma Scale as described above; localize any higher intracranial pathology; and assess brain-stem function.

Localize higher intracranial pathology

- Examine carefully for neck stiffness, and be aware that this becomes more difficult to detect with increasing depth of coma.
- Look for abnormal power and tone in all limbs and check all reflexes. As with neck stiffness, this becomes more difficult as the depth of coma increases.

- Look for deformity, particularly the typical 'spastic' rigidity of a pyramidal tract lesion.
- Look for abnormal deviation of the head and/or the eyes to one side. Deviation *away* from the weaker side indicates a contralateral cortical lesion because of the decussation (in the brain-stem) of both pyramidal tract fibres controlling motor activity of the head and limbs and of the supranuclear fibres controlling lateral conjugate gaze. Deviation of the eyes *towards* the weaker side is indicative of a lesion involving the pyramidal tract in the brain-stem, particularly with lesions in the pons affecting the supranuclear ocular motor fibres below their decussation (e.g. in the region of the 6th nerve nucleus). This is because decussation of the supranuclear fibres controlling lateral conjugate gaze occurs at a higher level in the brain-stem than the decussation of pyramidal tract motor fibres.

Assess brain-stem function

This is often regarded as something of a 'mystery', but adopting the following systematic approach helps enormously. Note that many of these signs have deep prognostic significance, which is vitally important when talking to relatives and deciding on the appropriate 'ceiling of care' for the patient.

Respiratory rate and rhythm

Several abnormal patterns of respiration can be recognized in the comatose patient (Fig. 2.1):

- **Cheyne–Stokes respiration**. Sometimes referred to as 'periodic breathing', this classical crescendo/de-crescendo pattern of respiration is usually indicative of bilateral cortical damage, but hypoxaemia, a prolonged circulation time and pulmonary congestion all enhance the appearance. Cheyne–Stokes respiration implies bilateral dysfunction of neurologic structures, usually lying deep within the cerebral hemispheres or in the diencephalon. The pathology is rarely placed as low as the upper pons.

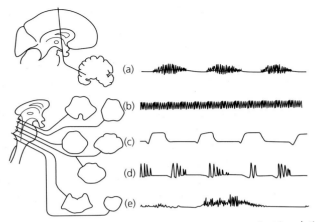

Fig. 2.1 Abnormal patterns of respiration in a comatose patient in relation to the anatomical site of the neurological pathology (see text): (a) Cheyne–Stokes respiration; (b) central neurogenic hyperventilation; (c) apneusis; (d) cluster breathing; (e) ataxic breathing. Reproduced with permission from Plum F and Posner JB, *The Diagnosis of Stupor and Coma*, 3rd edn (Oxford University Press, 2000)

It is frequently present in bilateral cerebral infarction and can accompany metabolic causes of coma, including hypertensive encephalopathy, uraemia and heart failure with cerebral hypoxia. The development of Cheyne–Stokes respiration in a comatose patient with a supratentorial mass lesion (including extensive haemorrhage) should suggest incipient transtentorial herniation.

- **Central neurogenic hyperventilation**. This pattern of respiratory abnormality occurs most commonly in patients with pathology affecting the low mid-brain to the middle third of the pons. It is quite rare: most cases of hyperpnoea in coma are either due to cardiopulmonary pathology or are secondary to metabolic acidosis.
- **Apneustic breathing**. A prolonged inspiratory phase is combined with a pause at full inspiration. Apneustic breathing is rare in humans; but a more common abnormality consisting of brief end-inspiratory pauses,

lasting 2–3 s and often alternating with end-expiratory pauses, is seen in basilar artery occlusion and occasionally in hypoglycaemia or even meningitis.

- **Cluster breathing**. This characteristic pattern (see Fig. 2.1) is not uncommon. It is a poor prognostic sign and usually indicates pathology in the lower pons or upper medulla.
- **Ataxic breathing**. This completely irregular pattern of breathing indicates disruption of the respiratory centre in the medulla oblongata. It is a grave prognostic sign and, importantly, is often accompanied by an exaggerated susceptibility of the respiratory centre to depressant drugs. Even mild sedation in patients with this respiratory rhythm can induce apnoea.

Pupils

The brain-stem areas controlling consciousness are anatomically adjacent to those controlling the pupils, so pupillary changes are a valuable guide to the presence and location of brain-stem pathology causing coma. Also, because the pupillary pathways are relatively resistant to metabolic insult, the presence or absence of the light reflex is a useful physical sign in distinguishing structural from metabolic coma.

Pupillary abnormalities in the comatose patient have potential value in localizing pathology.

- **Hypothalamic damage**. This can result in a unilateral Horner's syndrome, which can be the first sign of transtentorial herniation.
- **Mid-brain damage**. Pupils are often mid-point (5–6 mm in diameter), round, regular and fixed to light.
- **Pontine damage**. Lesions in the pons disrupt descending sympathetic pathways and produce bilaterally small pupils.
- **Lateral medullary and ventrolateral cervical cord lesions**. These often result in an ipsilateral Horner's syndrome.
- **Peripheral lesions**. Pupillary fibres in the 3rd nerve are particularly susceptible when uncal herniation compresses

the nerve against the posterior cerebral artery or the tentorial edge. In other words, lesions of the 3rd nerve close to its origin are likely to cause pupillary dilatation without accompanying extraocular ophthalmoplegias or ptosis. This is the 'blown pupil' and one should question either asymmetric tentorial herniation ('coning') or bleeding from a posterior communicating aneurysm.

- *In comparison*, lesions affecting the 3rd nerve more distally usually result in equal effects on the oculomotor and pupillomotor fibres.

The corneal reflex

Eyelids in comatose patients are usually closed but they are flaccid. If the eyelids are retracted manually in the truly comatose patient, they will drift back gradually to the closed position. In contrast, in *pseudocoma*, there will often be resistance to attempted movement of the eyelid by the examiner and when the eyelids are released they often shut with a snap!

- If corneal reflexes are absent in the deeply comatose patient the prognosis is very poor.
- If corneal reflexes are absent in a patient who is apparently in lighter coma, one should question drug intoxication, particularly opiate overdose.

Spontaneous eye movements

There are a few basic points to note.

- **Asymmetric oculomotor dysfunction** is more common with a structural brain lesion than with metabolic pathology.
- **Roving eye movements** are slow, random deviations of eye movement that are usually conjugate in nature. They are usually horizontal in direction but may be vertical. They indicate severe generalized cortical pathology, which may be structural or metabolic; and importantly, they cannot be mimicked by a patient presenting with pseudocoma.

- **Nystagmus** is rare in comatose patients because the quick phase of nystagmus relies on interaction between the oculovestibular system and the cerebral cortex. Nystagmus therefore disappears as cortical influence is reduced. However, there are rare variants of nystagmus that are useful in localizing pathology (see **Think** below).

> **THINK**
>
> Rare forms of nystagmus aid localization of pathology.
> - *Retractory nystagmus* refers to irregular jerking of the eyes back into the orbit, thought to be caused by contraction of all six ocular muscles at once. It is indicative of mesencephalic tegmental lesions.
> - *Convergence nystagmus* describes slow drifting of ocular divergence followed by a convergent jerk. It is usually due to a mid-brain lesion.
> - *Ocular bobbing* consists of intermittent, usually conjugate, brisk, downward eye movements. It is virtually pathognomonic of a severe destructive caudal pontine lesion.
> - *Nystagmoid jerking* of a single eye may be lateral, vertical or rotatory in nature and usually indicates severe mid to low pontine disease.

- **Abnormal conjugate deviation**. Deviation towards and away from a side of weakness has been discussed above, but be aware also of an irritative phenomenon that deviates the eyes away from the lesion. This can occur in cerebral haemorrhage, especially in the early stages, and may represent status epilepticus. Resting deviation of the eyes in a comatose patient below the midline is always indicative of brain-stem disease, although it can (reportedly) occur in hepatic encephalopathy.
- **Dysconjugate deviation**. A lesion of the 3rd nerve or its nucleus results in fixed pupillary dilatation and a divergent

eye ipsilaterally ('down and out'). A 6th nerve lesion results in an inward-looking eye.

- **Oculocephalic reflexes**. In light supratentorial coma, cortical influences are lost and movement of the head either laterally or 'up and down' results in 'doll's-eye' movements, by which the eyes maintain their original gaze. As coma deepens, the oculocephalic reflexes become brisker. In brain-stem pathology, these reflex movements are lost:
  - The mid-brain is responsible for maintaining upward gaze and pathology here will disrupt upward 'doll's eye' movements on vertical movement of the head.
  - Loss of lateral 'dolls-eye' movements implies disruption of the centre for lateral conjugate gaze and is therefore indicative of pathology affecting the lower pons or medulla.
- *Loss of oculocephalic reflexes is a poor prognostic sign in the comatose patient.*

● Investigations

Initial laboratory investigations

These are very important and are geared towards identifying potential causes of coma:

- blood sugar level
- full blood count, to look for evidence of sepsis
- clotting screen, to look for any evidence of a bleeding tendency
- renal function tests, to look for electrolyte disturbance
- liver function tests, to look for liver failure.

Also, investigate potential complications of the comatose state:

- chest radiograph, to look for aspiration pneumonia
- arterial blood gases, to assess for metabolic or respiratory acidosis
- plasma lactate.

Specific investigations

An investigation plan can be adequately constructed on the basis of categorizing the patient as follows.

Coma with focal brain-stem or localizing signs

Under these circumstances one is usually dealing with a tumour, an abscess, a bleed or an infarct. CT or MRI scanning is likely to be the definitive investigation. Occasionally this pattern of presentation can arise in metabolic coma (e.g. in hypoglycaemia) and rarely in hepatic encephalopathy.

Coma with no focal or localizing signs

Consider 'non-structural' or metabolic causes, such as:

- alcohol or drug overdose
- hypoxia
- hypothermia
- 'subtle' status epilepticus.

Investigate accordingly, including urgent electroencephalography (EEG) and consider specific therapeutic interventions as described below.

Coma with no focal or localizing signs but with neck stiffness

In this scenario, subarachnoid haemorrhage, meningitis and encephalitis are strong possibilities, so CT scanning, lumbar puncture and EEG must be considered urgently. Immediate antibiotics should be administered if meningitis is suspected and similarly antiviral therapy if there is any suggestion of herpes simplex encephalitis.

Identifying 'correctable coma'

This is an integral part of the investigation plan and it carries the highest priority. A continuing comatose state is accompanied by the potential for continuing brain damage, which may well be irreversible. In the following problem-solving approach we have included a series of clinical considerations, including a few classical pitfalls, under the **Think** and **Hazard** icons. Consider the following immediate possibilities *every time you see a comatose patient*.

- **Hypoglycaemia**. An immediate blood sugar estimation is mandatory. If you cannot get one, give 50 mL of 50% dextrose anyway and without delay.

HAZARD

Uncorrected hypoglycaemia causes neuroglycopaenia and progressive, potentially irreversible brain damage.

- **Opiate overdose**. Any feature suggestive of previous drug abuse or acute opiate toxicity (see **Think** below) is an indication for administration of naloxone. This is another example where the drug should be given on the slightest suspicion – but stand back after administering, because acute reversal of opiate toxicity often results in a violent response from the patient.

THINK

What are the specific signs of opiate toxicity?
They are: pin-point pupils; depressed respiration; hypotension; absent corneal reflexes when the consciousness level is not very reduced (GCS >5). This is probably because of the corneal anaesthetic effect of opiates.

- **Wernicke's encephalopathy**. Occasionally this can present with coma. Wernicke's encephalopathy is due to chronic alcohol abuse and is usually characterized by ataxia and ophthalmoplegias of various sorts. It can be associated with short-term memory loss combined with confabulation: Korsakoff's syndrome. It requires urgent treatment with thiamine; and if there is any suggestion of chronic alcohol abuse in the setting of coma then intravenous thiamine should be administered.

⚡ HAZARD

Chronic alcoholics are prone to hypoglycaemia as a result of alcohol-induced liver disease and, of course, glucose should be administered immediately to any alcoholic with hypoglycaemia. However, in this setting, thiamine must be administered concurrently because glucose on its own can induce acute Wernicke's encephalopathy.

- **Benzodiazepine overdose**. There is a specific antidote to benzodiazepine overdose, namely flumazenil. However, caution must be exercised when administering it (see **Hazard** below).

⚡ HAZARD .

Benzodiazepines are commonly taken as part of a mixed overdose which may contain tricyclic antidepressants. If the anticonvulsant effect of benzodiazepines is removed by administration of flumazenil, then the pro-convulsant effect of tricyclics can be unmasked and status epilepticus can result. Tricyclic-induced epilepsy carries a high mortality.

- **Non-convulsive status epilepticus**. This is covered also in Chapter 7. It exists when the continuing electrical seizure activity of the brain is no longer accompanied by recognizable motor activity. The best advice is to be very aware of this potential diagnosis in any comatose patient and especially in those who have a previous history of epilepsy. Look for the subtle clinical signs as mentioned earlier, seek help if there is any doubt, and empirical use of benzodiazepine may be justified.

- **Meningitis**. If there is any suggestion of meningitis, antibiotics must be administered with no delay. There are several diagnostic considerations to be aware of.

⚡ HAZARD

- As conscious level falls, the classical signs of meningism become more difficult to detect. A patient with a GCS of 5 as a result of bacterial meningitis may not manifest neck stiffness, for example.

- The rash of meningococcal septicaemia can be subtle in the early stages of the disease, and the advent of septicaemia (which is responsible for the skin rash) may lag behind that of meningeal infection. Look for a rash in the areas where it will first develop – this is commonly at pressure points. Turn the patient over and conscientiously examine the buttocks, backs of the thighs, extensor aspect of the arms and the elbows. These are areas that one may not automatically take in during a routine general examination.

- **Encephalitis**. The diagnosis of herpes simplex (HSV) encephalitis is easier if it is thought of! Consider it in any patient with a reduced conscious level for which no obvious reason can be found. The classical story is that of general symptoms constituting a prodrome for 12–24 hours before reduced consciousness follows. On examination, low to moderate fever is commonly present, there is a reduced GCS (but often not markedly so), the patient is 'irritable' and resents interference, and there may be signs of meningism. However, each or all of these classical presenting features may be absent. Think of the possibility and have a low threshold for administering antiviral therapy while a definitive diagnosis is made with CT, lumbar puncture, MRI and/or EEG investigations. All of these take time to arrange, but antiviral agents are more effective when administered early and they rarely cause adverse effects. The safest option, therefore, is to treat on suspicion of a diagnosis of HSV encephalitis.

- **Other correctable causes**. Although these conditions are unlikely causes of coma they are potentially correctable and are worthy of consideration:
  - hypothyroidism ('myxoedema coma'): very rare these days but with a high mortality risk
  - Addison's disease, which demands immediate fluid and steroid replacement (Addisonian crises are not uncommon in emergency departments but they rarely cause coma)
  - anaphylaxis: exactly the same comments apply.

3 Chest pain

● Introduction

The symptom of chest pain encompasses a spectrum from imminently life-threatening conditions at one extreme to 'benign' causes such as anxiety at the other. Many patients equate chest pain of any sort with potentially serious heart disease and anxiety often (understandably) complicates the presentation. A systematic approach to assessment of the patient can rule potentially life-threatening causes in or out fairly quickly. There will be some overlap in this chapter with Chapter 4 as the symptoms of chest pain and breathlessness often coexist.

> **HAZARD**
>
> Many students and junior medical staff think immediately of pulmonary embolism (PE) when seeing a patient with pleuritic chest pain. Although PE is undoubtedly a potential cause in some cases, alternative (and common) diagnoses are often overlooked. Many patients undergo unnecessary CT pulmonary angiography as a result, entailing significant radiation exposure. Most life-threatening PEs do not actually present with pleuritic chest pain – they are more likely to cause central chest pain and/or breathlessness. A careful risk assessment of the probability of a PE must be undertaken before requesting a CT pulmonary angiogram (see Table 3.1 for further information).

● Classification of chest pain

Potentially life-threatening causes of chest pain

Chest pain from these causes is usually central in site:

- Myocardial infarction (MI)
- Acute coronary syndrome (ACS)
- Massive pulmonary embolism (PE)
- Dissection of the thoracic aorta
- Tension pneumothorax
- Oesophageal rupture

Other causes of central chest pain are:

- Acute pericarditis
- Gastro-oesophageal reflux (GORD)
- Recreational drug use
  - Cocaine (may cause an acute coronary syndrome)
  - Amphetamines
- Anxiety

Causes of pleuritic type chest pain

Pain emanating from the pleura or chest wall and usually exacerbated by movement and coughing:

- Pulmonary embolism (PE) – usually smaller and more peripheral than those causing central chest pain
- Pneumonia
- Viral pleuritis (sometimes known as 'epidemic pleurodynia') – for example due to Coxsackie virus
- Pneumothorax
- Pleural empyema
- Chest trauma
- Rib fracture
- Rib metastases
- Malignant chest wall invasion by primary or secondary lung tumour
- Mesothelioma

- Multi-system inflammatory diseases
  - Rheumatoid arthritis (note however that, although episodes of pleuritic chest pain can occur in association with RA, rheumatoid pleural effusions are usually painless)
  - Systemic lupus erythematosus
- Pericarditis (note that the pain of pericarditis can vary, mimicking either cardiac chest pain or pleuritic chest pain)

THINK

What is pleurisy?
The term is not a diagnosis but a description of pleuritic chest pain. Patients often report an episode of pleurisy in their past medical history and the differential diagnosis of this event will be broad, as discussed above.

● History

Speed of onset

- A rapid onset of pain implies a cause that evolves quickly. Examples include myocardial infarct (MI), acute coronary syndrome (ACS), pulmonary embolism, aortic dissection, pneumothorax and rib fracture. The pleuritic chest pain of pneumonia can also have a surprisingly rapid onset. Always consider spontaneous pneumothorax in tall young men with sudden onset of pleuritic chest pain – although this is not an exclusive group for suffering this condition.
- Chest wall pain precipitated by a coughing fit may be caused by a 'cough fracture' of a rib. This usually occurs in elderly osteoporotic patients in whom minimal trauma is sufficient to result in fracture.

- Insidious onset of persistent chest wall pain is suspicious for malignancy such as mesothelioma or a peripheral lung tumour, which is invading the chest wall. Note that the lung itself does not contain pain fibres, so invasion of other structures (e.g. parietal pleura, nerves, intercostal muscles or ribs) is required for primary lung cancer to cause pain.

Character of the pain

- The pain of MI or ACS is typically central and 'heavy' or 'crushing' in nature. Patients often clench their fists over their chests when describing it.
- Aortic dissection classically causes a 'tearing' pain which radiates posteriorly between the scapulae.
- Gastro-oesophageal reflux disease (GORD) may cause a burning retrosternal pain but can be indistinguishable from cardiac-sounding pain.
- Pericarditis causes pain that is classically relieved by sitting forward. If the pain is located in the chest wall, sharper in nature and exacerbated by movement or coughing then it is 'pleuritic'. Note that not all causes of pleuritic chest pain originate in the pleura.

Radiation

- Radiation down the left arm (occasionally both arms) and especially to the lower jaw is suggestive of cardiac chest pain. The word 'angina' is actually derived from Greek meaning 'to choke'.
- As already mentioned, the pain of aortic dissection radiates through to the back between the scapulae.

Associated symptoms

- Some nausea and sweating is common with cardiac chest pain.
- Chest pain due to anxiety may be accompanied by associated symptoms of hyperventilation such as tingling extremities, light-headedness or a frank panic attack.

Periodicity

- Cardiac chest pain may have recurred in preceding weeks during exertion. A consistent history of recurrent exertional chest pain which resolves on rest requires urgent investigation for ischaemic heart disease.
- Chest pain that varies in intensity, site and onset may indicate anxiety. Typically there is no identifiable pattern to the precipitating factors and pain at rest is common.

Patient demographics and past medical history

- In the case of central chest pain, assess the patient for risk factors for ischaemic heart disease: diabetes, hypertension, hypercholesterolaemia, smoking, obesity, and a family history of premature ischaemic heart disease (with onset under the age of 60). In younger patients, consider recreational drug use and ask particularly about cocaine and amphetamines as these can cause coronary vasospasm.
- Major risk factors for PE include active malignancy, past history of confirmed venous thromboembolism, recent immobility, recent lower limb fracture or surgery, inherited thrombophilic disorders, pregnancy, or puerperium in women. Table 3.1 gives a summary

Table 3.1 Modified Wells criteria for assessing the risk of a pulmonary embolism in a patient presenting with symptoms suggestive of a possible PE

Clinical parameter	Score
Clinical evidence of DVT	3
No alternative diagnosis likely other than PE	3
Heart rate >100/min	1.5
Surgery or immobility in preceding 4 weeks	1.5
Previous confirmed DVT or PE	1.5
Haemoptysis	1
Active malignancy	1
Total score:	*Risk of a PE:*
>6	High: 78%
2–6	Moderate: 27%
<2	Low: 3.4%

DVT, deep vein thrombosis; PE, pulmonary embolism

of the modified Wells criteria that can be used to calculate the risk of a PE.

- If there is a history of insidious onset of intractable chest wall pain, consider a malignant cause and ascertain whether there is a history of:
  - a malignancy that has a propensity to metastasize to bone (in particular lung, prostate, breast, thyroid, renal)
  - asbestos exposure, since significant past exposure to asbestos may raise the possibility of mesothelioma (see **Think** below).

THINK

How can one reliably elicit a history of asbestos exposure? Many patients will readily recall occupational asbestos exposure but some may not, even in the face of evidence such as chest x-ray changes typical of asbestos exposure. Occupations with a high risk of exposure during the 1950s to 1980s include building, plumbing, carpentry, shipbuilding, railway carriage and power station construction, insulation, and service on naval ships. 'DIY' home renovations have also entailed a risk of exposure in some countries, notably Australia where asbestos was mined and used extensively in home construction during the 1950s to 1970s. The time lag between exposure and subsequent lung or pleural pathology is over 20 years.

Trauma

- If the pain is pleuritic in nature, ask about chest trauma. In frail elderly patients or those with risk factors for osteoporosis, ask whether the onset occurred during a coughing fit, as this may indicate a cough fracture. The typical patient with a cough fracture will be an elderly patient with chronic obstructive pulmonary disease (COPD) who has been on prolonged oral corticosteroid therapy. If significant breathlessness is a feature in the context of a possible rib fracture, then traumatic pneumothorax is a possibility.

- Chest pain occurring after copious vomiting or after any form of medical intervention involving upper gastrointestinal endoscopy may raise the possibility of oesophageal rupture. This has a high mortality if not promptly recognized and treated.

Symptoms of infection

- In the case of pleuritic type chest pain, fever, cough and 'flu-like symptoms increase the likelihood of pneumonia or viral pleuritis.
- Headache is common in pneumonia.

● Examination

The potentially life-threatening causes of chest pain listed above may lead to haemodynamic instability and shock, so the first parameters to check on examination are:

- pulse rate
- blood pressure
- respiratory rate
- oxygen saturation.

Note also whether the patient appears pale, clammy, grey or cyanosed – any of which can indicate a potentially life-threatening situation. If the patient is shocked or hypotensive, then immediate attention will be required with regard to the airway, intravenous access, fluid resuscitation and oxygen administration. Urgent investigations including an electro-cardiogram and chest x-ray will be needed before completing a full examination.

If the patient is stable, then it is safe to proceed with a full examination with particular attention to the following.

- **Jugular venous pressure**. In the context of central chest pain, a raised JVP may indicate acutely raised right ventricular pressure due to a PE, or biventricular cardiac failure.
- **Radial pulses and blood pressure**. Look for inequalities between the radial pulses and blood pressure in each arm, as this can be a sign of aortic dissection.
- **Tracheal deviation**. If present, this could indicate either a tension pneumothorax (in which case the trachea is pushed away from the pneumothorax) or a less severe large pneumothorax (in which case the trachea can be pushed over towards the pneumothorax by overexpansion of the normal lung).
- **Heart sounds**. Listen carefully for murmurs or a pericardial rub. Aortic stenosis can, for example, cause angina. A pericardial rub is a diagnostic sign of pericarditis but can be intermittent, so absence of a rub does not rule out the diagnosis.
- **Chest percussion**. Dullness in one lower zone (with reduced or absent breath sounds) and associated with chest pain may indicate a pleural effusion. Causes of a pleural effusion in the context of chest pain include pneumonia, empyema, PE, chest trauma (haemothorax), malignancy and multi-system inflammatory diseases. Hyper-resonance may indicate the presence of a pneumothorax, although in practice this is a subtle and difficult sign to elicit.
- **Breath sounds**. Bilateral basal crackles may indicate left ventricular failure, which can occur following an MI or ACS. Note, however, that crackles can also be a feature of other respiratory pathology such as pulmonary fibrosis or alveolitis. In addition the absence of crackles does not exclude a diagnosis of cardiac failure. Focal crackles or

bronchial breathing can occur in pneumonia. A pleural rub is a marker of pleural inflammation and can occur in viral pleuritis, pneumonia, peripheral PE and multi-system inflammatory diseases. Just like pericardial rubs, pleural rubs can be intermittent. Reduced or absent breath sounds with a dull percussion note may indicate a pleural effusion.

- **Chest wall tenderness**. Localized pain on palpation can indicate a soft tissue injury, rib fracture, rib metastasis or malignant invasion of chest wall structures.

● Investigations

Some simple initial investigations should be performed without delay in any patient presenting with chest pain. These will enable some potentially life-threatening conditions to be diagnosed or excluded quickly.

Electrocardiography (ECG)

There are particular patterns of abnormality to look for.

- With ST segment elevation MI, prompt treatment with thrombolysis or primary angioplasty may be indicated.
- ST segment depression indicates coronary ischaemia.
- Sinus tachycardia and non-specific ST segment changes are the commonest ECG findings in most cases of PE, which are not massive or immediately life-threatening (see **Hazard** below).
- Right axis deviation with complete or partial right bundle branch block may indicate acute right ventricular strain from a larger and more potentially life-threatening PE.
- The 'S1 Q3 T3' triad of findings classically described in every textbook comprises an S wave in lead 1, Q wave in lead 3 and inverted T wave in lead 3. It denotes acute severe right ventricular overload due to a massive PE.

Most patients with this ECG finding will be shocked and extremely unwell (see **Hazard** below).

- 'Concave upward' ST elevation is typical of acute pericarditis.

HAZARD

Many junior medical staff assume that the 'S1 Q3 T3' pattern of abnormality can be found in any case of PE. This is not the case. Remember that the most common ECG abnormalities in PE are a sinus tachycardia and non-specific ST segment changes. 'S1 Q3 T3' is seen only in massive PE causing acute severe right ventricular strain. Note that it is neither a sensitive nor a specific finding for PE and in the opinion of the authors it is overrated as a diagnostic tool for PE.

Chest x-ray (CXR)

Patterns of abnormality that should help in narrowing the differential diagnosis on a reasonable quality CXR include the following.

- If the mediastinum is widened on a good-quality posteroanterior (PA) CXR, then aortic dissection must be considered in the differential diagnosis of acute central chest pain. Aortic dissection is, however, still possible in the absence of mediastinal widening, and the only reliable way to exclude it, if clinically suspected, is with a contrast-enhanced CT scan of the thorax. Note that an anteroposterior (AP) film will not enable you to assess the width of the mediastinum adequately as it will appear artificially widened.
- Pneumothorax should be readily diagnosed (or ruled out) on a CXR (Fig. 3.1). Be aware of the risk of mistaking a large bulla on the CXR of an emphysematous patient for a

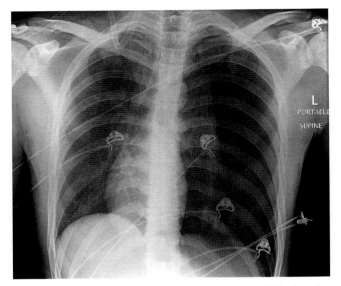

Fig. 3.1 Large left-sided tension pneumothorax. Note the shift of the heart and mediastinum to the right, away from the pneumothorax, indicating that it is under tension

pneumothorax. Inserting a chest drain into a bulla may have disastrous consequences.

- Most rib fractures should be clearly visible on a good-quality CXR. Sometimes chest pain prevents the patient inhaling fully, which can result in a fracture in a lower rib being obscured by soft tissue.

- Focal shadowing or consolidation indicates pneumonia. Absolutely clear lung fields exclude the diagnosis of pneumonia.

- A malignant tumour causing rib destruction should be readily visible as peripheral shadowing.

- A small pleural reaction or blunting of one costophrenic angle indicates possible viral pleuritis or a PE.

- An area of band atelectasis with a slightly elevated hemidiaphragm, particularly in association with a blunt

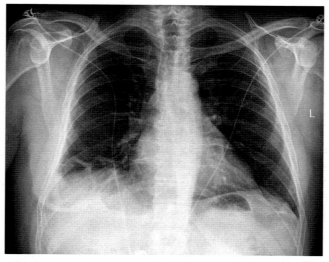

Fig. 3.2 Chest x-ray study in a patient with extensive pulmonary emboli on computerized tomography (CT) pulmonary angiogram. Note the two band shadows and blunt costophrenic angle at the right base

costophrenic angle, is suspicious for a PE (Fig. 3.2) (see **Think** below).

- A moderate-sized pleural effusion, depending on the clinical picture, may indicate underlying pneumonia (a 'parapneumonic effusion'), pleural empyema, PE, malignancy, haemothorax, mesothelioma or multi-system inflammatory disease.

THINK

What are the common CXR findings in PE?
The classical textbook description of a 'wedge-shaped infarct' is actually rare. Over 90 per cent of patients with a proven PE have abnormalities on their initial CXR, many of which are seemingly minor and often overlooked.

Common patterns of abnormality in PE include a small pleural effusion, a pleural reaction manifesting as a blunt costophrenic angle, and areas of subsegmental atelectasis. A larger PE may produce an area of oligaemia in one lung (known as Westermark's sign), perhaps in association with a proximal bulky pulmonary artery. In addition, a larger pleural effusion or lobar pulmonary infarct similar in appearance to lobar pneumonia may be seen.

Laboratory tests

These should be tailored to the presentation, but many cases will require the following.

- *Full blood count.* Look for anaemia (which may precipitate cardiac ischaemia and chest pain) and a raised neutrophil count if infection such as pneumonia or empyema is suspected.
- *Serum C-reactive protein* (CRP). This is typically elevated to over 250 mg/L in pneumonia and empyema.
- *Urea and electrolytes.* In the case of suspected cardiac ischaemia, serum potassium levels should be kept above 4 mmol/L to reduce the risk of myocardial irritability. A serum urea level above 7 mmol/L is a poor prognostic feature in acute pneumonia.
- *Cardiac troponin level.* This should be measured in all cases of central chest pain, at least 12 hours after the onset of pain. It is raised in MI and can be raised in ACS and notably PE (due to acute right ventricular strain). It is also raised in chronic renal failure (owing to impaired renal excretion of troponin) and in sepsis; so caution must be exercised in interpreting the result in a patient with these conditions.
- *D-dimer.* This test is useful only in differential diagnosis if it is negative in a patient who is at low risk for a PE, in which case a PE is effectively ruled out. A positive D-dimer has low

specificity, with its many potential causes including recent surgery, immobility and recent illness. If a patient with chest pain is at moderate or high risk for a PE (see Table 3.1 on p. 36), then a CT pulmonary angiogram or ventilation/perfusion lung scan to look for a PE is indicated and a D-dimer test adds nothing to the diagnostic process.

- *Serum calcium level.* This is indicated if a malignant cause is suspected for chest wall pain. An elevated serum calcium is fairly common in the presence of bone metastases, and requires prompt treatment.

Further radiological investigations

Depending on the individual presentation, further imaging may be required.

- If aortic dissection is suspected, obtain a CT of the thorax with intravenous contrast (Fig. 3.3).
- If PE is suspected, do a CT pulmonary angiogram (CTPA) or ventilation/perfusion (V/Q) scan. If a massive PE is

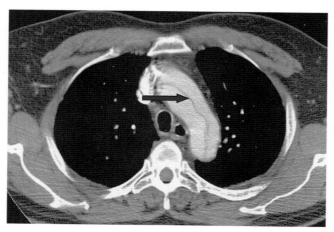

Fig. 3.3 Computerized tomography of the thorax with contrast showing aortic dissection. Note the 'double lumen' in the aortic arch caused by the dissected vessel wall (arrowed)

suspected in a shocked patient, an echocardiogram is the immediate investigation of choice (see **Think** below).

- If an empyema is suspected, obtain a CT of the thorax to assess the possible need for surgical drainage. An urgent opinion from a respiratory physician or thoracic surgeon should be sought regarding management.
- If a malignant cause for chest pain is suspected, obtain a CT of the thorax followed by a specialist opinion from a respiratory physician regarding management.

THINK

Which is the better test for a suspected pulmonary embolism, CTPA or V/Q?
In most cases CTPA gives a more reliable result and international guidelines on PE management usually recommend a CTPA as the investigation of choice. V/Q scans are difficult to interpret in the presence of chronic lung disease and should not be requested in patients with COPD or pulmonary fibrosis, for example. In addition, V/Q scans in patients with moderate PE risk have poor sensitivity and specificity. The radiation dose from a CTPA (~400 CXRs), however, far exceeds that from a V/Q scan (~65 CXRs), and in some circumstances – such as pregnancy – a V/Q scan may be a safer option.

THINK

How can one quickly confirm a diagnosis of PE in a shocked patient who is too unwell to be moved to a CT scanning department?
Request an urgent echocardiogram, which can be performed at the patient's bedside. The presence of acute right ventricular strain can confirm the diagnosis sufficiently for thrombolytic agents to be administered.

CLINICAL TIP

Some causes of chest pain, such as GORD and anxiety, are diagnoses of exclusion. If no significant cause has been identified for ongoing chest pain, then administering a dose of antacid is an acceptable course of action, to see whether the pain is partially or wholly relieved. A 'therapeutic trial' in this way may aid diagnosis.

4 Breathlessness

● Introduction

Occasional breathlessness is a universal human experience. Reporting breathlessness as a symptom is often about context and the perception of the patient as to whether the degree of breathlessness being experienced is appropriate or not. Breathlessness may be a normal sensation in healthy people after exercise, it may reflect a lack of fitness in an overweight individual who perceives himself as abnormally breathless compared with his peers, or it may be symptomatic of serious pathology.

The differential diagnosis of breathlessness is broad and in this chapter we offer a systematic approach to separating the 'groups' of diagnoses listed in a logical fashion. A separate section of the chapter is dedicated to 'breathlessness with wheeze' as this encompasses a distinct group of differential diagnoses.

Because breathlessness and chest pain commonly coexist there is some inevitable overlap with Chapter 3.

● Classification of breathlessness

Pulmonary and thoracic origin

- Small airways disease
  - Asthma
  - Chronic obstructive pulmonary disease
  - Anaphylaxis
  - Bronchiectasis – if there is associated airflow obstruction and wheezing
- Large airways disease
  - Stridor, caused by partial obstruction of the trachea or major airway
  - Lobar collapse due to obstruction by tumour, mucus plug or foreign body
- Infection
  - Pneumonia, usually bacterial, can be viral (10% of cases)
  - Bronchitis, usually viral
  - Pneumonitis, usually viral
  - Tuberculosis
  - HIV-associated (e.g. pneumocystis pneumonia)
- Interstitial lung disease
  - Idiopathic pulmonary fibrosis (commonly referred to as 'cryptogenic fibrosing alveolitis' or by its histological classification of 'usual interstitial pneumonia')
  - Sarcoidosis
  - Asbestosis/pneumoconiosis
  - Acute alveolitis/hypersensitivity pneumonitis (many allergens can be responsible, e.g. bird-fancier's lung and farmers' lung)
  - Drug-induced
  - Pulmonary vasculitis
- Pleural disease
  - Pneumothorax
  - Pleural effusion

- Bilateral (usually transudative): common causes are cardiac failure and hypoproteinaemic states
- Unilateral (usually exudative): common causes are malignancy, pneumonia (including empyema) and PE; a less common cause of a left-sided effusion is pancreatitis
- Pleural thickening/fibrosis
- Mesothelioma
- Pulmonary vascular disease
  - Pulmonary embolism (PE)
  - Pulmonary hypertension – which can be primary ('idiopathic') or secondary
- Respiratory muscle weakness
  - Diaphragm paralysis due to phrenic nerve palsy or Guillain–Barré syndrome, for example
  - Neuromuscular disease such as motor neurone disease, muscular dystrophy
- Chest wall disease
  - Severe scoliosis
  - Extensive previous thoracic wall surgery such as thoracoplasty (this is no longer performed)

Cardiac origin
- Left ventricular failure leading to pulmonary oedema
- Ischaemic heart disease
- Cardiomyopathy:
  - Alcoholic cardiomyopathy
  - Viral cardiomyopathy
  - Ischaemic cardiomyopathy
- Valvular heart disease
- Constrictive pericardial disease (TB and rheumatoid)
- Pericardial effusion, particularly of malignant origin
- Arrhythmias
  - Atrial fibrillation
  - Heart block: second- and third-degree

Metabolic causes
- Acute metabolic acidosis
  - Diabetic ketoacidosis
  - Acute renal failure
  - Lactic acidosis
  - Salicylate poisoning
- Anaemia
- Hypothyroidism

Miscellaneous
- Hyperventilation syndrome
- Obesity or lack of fitness

THINK

What are the causes of pulmonary hypertension?
Most cases of pulmonary hypertension (PHT) are
secondary to chronic lung disease such as chronic
obstructive pulmonary disease (COPD) or pulmonary
fibrosis, when it is commonly referred to as *cor pulmonale*.
Less common causes of secondary PHT include:
- severe obstructive sleep apnoea or obesity
  hypoventilation syndrome
- chronic thromboembolic PHT (CTEPH)
- congenital heart disease with right–left shunt
  (Eisenmenger's syndrome)
- severe mitral stenosis
- sarcoidosis – usually only in chronic and severe cases
- HIV infection
- multi-system inflammatory diseases such as systemic
  lupus erythematosis (SLE)
- chronic ingestion of stimulants such as amphetamines
  and cocaine.

Some cases have no identifiable cause and are termed
'idiopathic', although some mechanisms of causation are
now being identified at a molecular level.

HAZARD

Beware of the possibility of 'silent angina' in patients describing consistent exertional breathlessness with no chest pain. In some patients, coronary artery disease presents only with breathlessness on exertion and a treadmill exercise test may reveal typical ischaemic changes on ECG but with no accompanying chest pain.

● History

Your approach to taking a history will need to be tailored to the urgency of the clinical situation. An acutely breathless patient in an emergency department may be too breathless to speak much and the history will need to be brief. Further history can be obtained once the patient has recovered sufficiently to be questioned in more detail. On the other hand, a detailed history is particularly important in the context of interstitial lung disease because of the variety of its potential causes. In an outpatient setting there is more time to explore all aspects of the history carefully (e.g. occupational exposure). As always, focused questioning assists in the differential diagnosis.

Speed of onset

- This provides vital information. A rapid onset (minutes to hours) usually indicates rapidly evolving pathology such as acute pulmonary oedema, anaphylaxis, acute asthma, pneumothorax, pulmonary embolism, acute metabolic acidosis or a cardiac arrhythmia.
- Slower onset (hours to days) is more common with most infections, exacerbations of COPD and some forms of acute interstitial lung disease (e.g. acute alveolitis).
- Even slower onset (days to weeks) is seen in pleural effusions, lobar collapse, anaemia, cardiomyopathy, tuberculosis, pneumocystis pneumonia and respiratory muscle weakness.

- Insidious onset (weeks to months and more) is seen in tuberculosis, valvular heart disease, many forms of interstitial lung disease (pulmonary fibrosis is the best example), pleural thickening, mesothelioma, pulmonary hypertension and chest wall abnormalities. A history of insidious onset over years is not unusual in pulmonary fibrosis and pulmonary hypertension.

Orthopnoea

Most causes of breathlessness are exacerbated by lying supine (orthopnoea), but pulmonary oedema and respiratory muscle weakness are particular causes of orthopnoea. The converse of orthopnoea is *platypnoea*, breathlessness that is worse on sitting up. This (often overlooked) symptom is typical of a major pulmonary embolism, when lying supine improves venous return to the heart and increases cardiac output, thereby decreasing the sensation of breathlessness.

Cough

A non-productive ('dry') cough is common in interstitial lung disease, pneumonia and with central airway occluding tumours. A weak or absent cough is suspicious for neuromuscular disease. Particular associations with a *productive* cough include the following.

- There is sputum production in small airways diseases such as asthma, COPD and bronchiectasis.
- There is production of frothy sputum in pulmonary oedema and the sputum may be tinged with blood.
- Haemoptysis can occur in pulmonary embolism, major airway lung tumours and pulmonary vasculitis. The classical textbook description of 'rusty sputum' in pneumococcal pneumonia is quite unusual. Blood-streaked sputum is fairly common in acute bronchitis and exacerbations of COPD, as a result of intense airway inflammation.

- A productive cough of more than three weeks' duration in a patient with risk factors for tuberculosis (TB) should raise suspicion for pulmonary TB. The main risk factors in developed countries are birth in a high-incidence country (see Chapter 16), immunosuppression and refugee status.

Wheeze

The presence of wheezing may narrow the differential diagnosis of breathlessness considerably. See the later section 'Breathlessness with wheeze'.

Associated symptoms

- **Chest pain**. Some cases of breathlessness may be associated with chest pain. Examples are central chest pain in ischaemic heart disease or a major PE, and pleuritic chest pain in pneumonia, pneumothorax and a smaller PE. Refer to Chapter 3 for more information.
- **Infection**. Fever with or without rigors suggests infection such as pneumonia. A headache is also common in pneumonia. A prolonged fever (more than two weeks) with weight loss and night sweats should raise suspicion of TB.

Exacerbating and relieving factors

Almost all cases of breathlessness are exacerbated by exertion and relieved by rest and this information is a poor discriminator of diagnoses. The notable exception is hyperventilation syndrome (HVS), which often causes breathlessness that is unpredictable and variable in intensity in similar situations.

> **THINK**
>
> *What are the features of hyperventilation syndrome?*
> Clues to the diagnosis include:
> - breathlessness with a sensation of being 'unable to take a deep enough breath'
> - breathlessness when talking, often on the phone

- unpredictable onset and variation in severity of symptoms
- accompanying tingling of the fingers or around the mouth, caused by a temporary reduction in ionized calcium due to respiratory alkalosis
- a history of anxiety or depression
- multiple other unexplained symptoms despite extensive investigations, for example abdominal pain, chest pain or headache
- normal investigations such as chest radiograph, ECG, lung function tests and echocardiogram
- oxygen saturation of 99–100 per cent on air (normal is usually around 95–98 per cent).

Risk factors for PE or ischaemic heart disease

A full description of these, together with the Wells criteria for assessing PE risk, can be found in Chapter 3.

Patient history

Smoking history

Quantifying the smoking history is important. Calculate the pack-years smoked (see **Think** box) as the risk of diseases such as COPD and lung cancer rises linearly with lifetime tobacco consumption. Ask also about cannabis smoking as cannabis is even more harmful to the lungs than tobacco.

THINK

How does one calculate pack-years of smoking?
First ask the patient at what age he or she started smoking and when/if they have quit. Then ask what the

average consumption was in cigarettes per day. The formula for calculating pack years is:

$$\text{Pack-years} = \frac{\text{no. of cigarettes per day}}{20} \times \text{no. of years of smoking}$$

If a patient has been a smoker of 'roll-up' tobacco or pipe tobacco, assume that 2 ounces (50 g) of tobacco per week is roughly equivalent to 20 cigarettes per day. A cannabis joint is equivalent to about five cigarettes, and a cigar is also roughly equivalent to about five cigarettes in terms of exposure to carcinogens. The risk of lung cancer and COPD rises linearly above about 20 pack-years of smoking.

Medical history

Some pre-existing medical history may have particular relevance in the context of new-onset breathlessness.

- **Cardiac or respiratory disease**. Although this will increase the likelihood that the current presentation is related to a pre-existing condition, don't assume that this is the case.
- **Diabetes**. Rapid-onset breathlessness can sometimes be the presenting feature of metabolic acidosis in diabetic ketoacidosis.
- **Malignancy**. Many tumours can metastasize to the pleura or pericardium and cause pleural or pericardial effusions. Pleural effusions due to breast and lung cancer are the most common examples. In addition, some chemotherapeutic agents can cause long-term side-effects such as cardiomyopathy or pulmonary fibrosis.
- **Multi-system inflammatory diseases**. Interstitial lung disease can occur in association with rheumatoid arthritis and SLE, for example.
- **Neuromuscular disease**. Respiratory muscle weakness can complicate conditions such as motor neurone disease and myotonic dystrophy.

Is HIV infection a possibility?

This must be considered in any new case of interstitial lung disease or suspected TB. See Chapter 16 for information on risk factors for HIV.

History of occupational exposure?

A detailed occupational history may be neither relevant nor feasible in an emergency situation, so the more detailed enquiry will need to be postponed to a later stage when the patient is clinically stable. Initial radiological investigations often raise the question of occupational lung disease.

- A detailed Think box on asbestos exposure can be found in Chapter 3 on p. 37.
- Did the patient work in the mining industry, particularly coal mining or gold mining in the era before improved occupational safety standards were introduced?
- Has there been exposure to agents that can cause hypersensitivity pneumonitis? These include mouldy hay in farming and flour in bakeries. A full list of the potential causative agents of hypersensitivity pneumonitis is beyond the scope of this text.
- Has there been exposure to agents or environments that may precipitate asthma attacks? Spray paints, glutaraldehyde or cold air in refrigerated premises are examples.

Drug history

This is particularly important if you suspect interstitial lung disease as a potential diagnosis. Many drugs are known to cause acute pneumonitis or pulmonary fibrosis. Amiodarone and methotrexate are two common examples, but a plethora of drugs may be responsible and, in any case of undiagnosed interstitial lung disease, it is safe practice to check every drug the patient has taken for a possible causative association. A specialist respiratory opinion is commonly required.

Pets

Again this is an important question in suspected interstitial lung disease. Ask particularly about exposure to birds, because many species are associated with hypersensitivity pneumonitis. Pigeon fanciers and keepers of psittacine (parrot family) birds are particularly at risk, but many other species have been described as causing the hypersensitivity pneumonitis of 'bird-fanciers' lung'.

Breathlessness with wheeze

Wheezing is a musical sound caused by narrowing of airways. Most causes result in widespread polyphonic wheezing on expiration produced from multiple narrowed airways of differing calibre. Wheeze (usually accompanied by breathlessness) is a common cause of presentation to emergency medical services. The two most common causes in adults are:

- acute severe asthma
- exacerbation of COPD.

Other less common causes of widespread polyphonic wheezing are:

- acute pulmonary oedema
- acute viral bronchitis
- pulmonary embolism
- exacerbation of bronchiectasis
- anaphylaxis.

Wheezing may also be localized and monophonic if it is generated from a single obstructed airway, and this can occur in larger airway obstruction caused by:

- tumour
- aspirated foreign body
- mucus plugging.

In these conditions the chest x-ray is likely to be abnormal and specialist respiratory referral is indicated.

● Examination

Breathlessness may indicate a potentially life-threatening diagnosis and, therefore, immediate assessment of the airway, vital signs and other respiratory indices must take precedence over the remainder of the examination in order to evaluate the acuity of the clinical situation.

- *Respiratory rate.* A rate >24/minute indicates the potential for developing respiratory failure and constitutes a medical emergency.
- *Pulse rate.* Tachycardia is common in many of the causes of breathlessness we have listed. Both a very high pulse rate (>120/min) and a low pulse rate can indicate increasing severity of disease. Bradycardia may indicate the presence of heart block. In the context of an acute respiratory illness such as asthma or pneumonia, bradycardia indicates a life-threatening degree of severity.
- *Blood pressure.* Hypotension in the context of breathlessness usually indicates haemodynamic compromise and is a medical emergency.
- *Use of accessory muscles of respiration.* When present (often in the context of asthma or COPD) this is indicative of a severe exacerbation.

- *Oxygen saturation.* Note whether the patient is breathing air or oxygen.
- *Central cyanosis.* Note that this can be an unreliable sign, because the absence of cyanosis does not rule out respiratory failure.

THINK

Why is cyanosis an unreliable sign?
At least 5 g/L of deoxygenated haemoglobin must be circulating for cyanosis to be evident. In an anaemic patient, for example, with a haemoglobin level of 8 g/L this will not be possible (as it would probably be incompatible with life). Conversely in a polycythaemic patient with a haemoglobin level of 18 g/L cyanosis can be present even in the absence of any respiratory disease or tissue hypoxia.

- *Smell of ketones.* This may indicate diabetic ketoacidosis.

Differential diagnosis

Careful attention to the following examination findings will help to narrow the differential diagnosis. The details are summarized in Table 4.1.

Chest anatomy and expansion
Look for the barrel chest of emphysema, scars from previous surgery, and developmental malformations such as scoliosis. Is chest expansion symmetrical? Asymmetry is usually best observed from the end of the bed. Possible causes of asymmetry include lobar collapse or pneumothorax. Patients with scoliosis or extensive previous chest wall surgery will have asymmetrical expansion at all times.

Jugular venous pressure
If JVP is elevated, consider biventricular cardiac failure, right heart failure due to PE, pulmonary hypertension, cor pulmonale or pericardial disease.

Table 4.1 Summary of signs on examination in common respiratory conditions

	Trachea	Expansion	Percussion note	Vocal fremitus	Breath sounds	Clubbing
Pneumothorax	May be deviated	Reduced on affected side	Hyperresonant	Absent	Reduced/absent	No
Pneumonia	Central	Normal	Dull over affected area	Increased over affected area	Focal crackles or bronchial breathing (perhaps with whispering pectoriloquy)	No
Pleural effusion	Deviated away from effusion if massive	Normal	Dull or 'stony' dull	Absent	Reduced/absent	Possible in lung cancer or empyema
Pleural thickening	Central	Normal	Dull	Normal	Reduced	No
Lobar collapse	Deviated towards lesion	Reduced on affected side	Usually normal	Normal	Usually normal	Possible in lung cancer
Diaphragm paralysis	Central	Reduced on affected side	Dull at base	Absent	Reduced/absent	No
Asthma/COPD	Central	Reduced: hyperexpanded chest	Normal	Normal	Wheeze, often focal crackles in COPD	No
Bronchiectasis	Central	Normal	Usually normal	Normal	Focal crackles and often wheeze	Possible
Cardiac failure (LVF)	Central	Normal	May be dull at bases	May be reduced at bases	Crackles	No
Pulmonary fibrosis	Central	Reduced globally	Normal	Normal	Crackles	Possible
Acute alveolitis/ pneumonitis	Central	Normal	Normal	Normal	Crackles, which may be subtle	No

COPD, chronic obstructive pulmonary disease; LVF, left ventriular failure

Tracheal deviation

Deviation indicates a significant shift of mediastinal structures and usually implies gross pathology. Remember that deviation will be towards the side of the lesion in lobar collapse or a pneumothorax without tension. Conversely deviation will be away from the lesion in a tension pneumothorax or massive pleural effusion.

Percussion note

Basal dullness may indicate an effusion, substantial pleural thickening or a raised hemidiaphragm (e.g. due to diaphragm paralysis). Attention to other examination findings (such as breath sounds and vocal fremitus) will be necessary in order to elucidate the reason for dullness to percussion. Although a hyperresonant percussion note is classically described in pneumothorax, this is difficult to detect in practice, particularly if there is a lot of background noise.

Breath sounds

Note the location of any abnormal breath sounds. Particular patterns to look for include the following.

Inspiratory crackles

If crackles are detected, ask the patient to cough and repeat your auscultation.

- Persistent bilateral unchanging crackles indicate pulmonary oedema, alveolar inflammation ('alveolitis') or pulmonary fibrosis.
- In advanced pulmonary fibrosis you may hear classical 'Velcro' type crackles.
- Focal crackles are common in pneumonia.
- Crackles that change or disappear after coughing indicate the presence of sputum (commonly in COPD and bronchiectasis) or atelectasis from prolonged immobility.

Noisy breathing

- Expiratory wheeze usually indicates small airways disease as a result of asthma or COPD, but there are some other less common causes as described earlier.
- Stridor has been described earlier (see **Hazard** on p. 59).

Reduced or absent breath sounds

This suggests the presence of pleural effusion, pneumothorax or gross pleural thickening.

Bronchial breathing

Bronchial breathing is the cardinal sign of lung consolidation and a very satisfying sign to find! It is not common in pneumonia – localized crackles are more common. It may be associated with increased vocal fremitus (see below) or whispering pectoriloquy. The latter is present when the patient is asked to whisper and the transmitted sounds appear to be in the examiner's head rather than at the diaphragm end of the stethoscope.

Pleural rubs

A pleural rub indicates pleural inflammation from any cause and may be present in pneumonia, peripheral PE, viral pleuritis and multi-system inflammatory diseases. As described in Chapter 3, pleural rubs can be both transient and intermittent.

Vocal fremitus

Tactile vocal fremitus involves detecting the vibration of speech at the chest wall. It will be absent if air (pneumothorax) or fluid (effusion) are present to dampen the vibration. The same information is gained by means of using vocal resonance: the patient speaks and the examiner listens with a stethoscope for transmitted sounds. Vocal resonance is reduced by both pleural fluid and pneumothorax. Although the combination of a dull percussion note and reduced vocal fremitus and resonance is typical of a pleural effusion, remember that a raised hemidiaphragm can produce the same combination of signs.

HAZARD

It is easy to assume that a dull basal percussion note with reduced or absent breath sounds and reduced vocal fremitus is indicative of a pleural effusion, but the same signs can indicate diaphragm paralysis. Before attempting pleurocentesis always obtain a chest x-ray in order to avoid inserting a needle inadvertently into the patient's liver or spleen.

Heart sounds
Listen carefully for murmurs or signs of cardiac failure such as a gallop rhythm.

Clubbing
Finger clubbing is associated with a number of pathologies. It is an insensitive sign and its absence does not exclude any of the following:

- longstanding idiopathic pulmonary fibrosis
- lung cancer
- chronic intrathoracic sepsis such as bronchiectasis or empyema
- familial idiopathic clubbing (always ask the patient if the nail appearances are a new finding).

Ankle swelling
Bilateral ankle oedema in the context of breathlessness may indicate biventricular cardiac failure or pulmonary hypertension (cor pulmonale in the presence of known COPD or other chronic lung disease).

Abdominal paradox
If you suspect respiratory muscle weakness (e.g. in a patient with known neuromuscular disease) it is helpful to observe the movement of the abdominal wall during respiration lying supine. In a normal subject the abdominal wall should rise on

inspiration as the diaphragm descends and displaces abdominal contents. In significant respiratory muscle weakness the abdominal wall can be seen being sucked inwards as negative intrathoracic pressure during inspiration sucks the contents up with a paralysed diaphragm.

● Investigations

Many of the conditions listed as causes of breathlessness can be confirmed or excluded on fairly simple tests that can be performed in most emergency departments.

Laboratory tests

The following can be useful:

- full blood count to exclude anaemia
- cardiac troponins if acute pulmonary oedema is suspected
- blood glucose or finger-prick glucose if ketoacidosis is suspected
- urea and electrolytes if metabolic acidosis is suspected
- arterial blood gases if metabolic acidosis is suspected
- thyroid function tests (usually applicable with a long history in an outpatient setting).

Brain natriuretic peptide (BNP) may be indicated when cardiac failure is suspected but not clinically evident or not confirmed on other simple investigations such as a chest x-ray. It is not indicated if other evidence of cardiac failure is present.

Radiological investigations

Chest radiograph

This will usually confirm or raise strong suspicion of the following conditions, but further imaging or confirmatory investigations will often be required to achieve a precise diagnosis:

- acute pulmonary oedema
- pneumonia

- pneumothorax
- interstitial lung disease (note that 10 per cent of cases are not evident on a plain CXR)
- pleural effusion
- lobar collapse
- pulmonary TB
- pneumocystis pneumonia
- bronchiectasis (although this is frequently not seen on a plain CXR)
- pleural thickening
- mesothelioma.

Note that the chest x-ray is often normal or unremarkable in asthma and COPD, although hyperinflated lungs may be present and emphysematous bullae may be seen in COPD.

Chest CT

This will be indicated in the following situations. Note that several different CT protocols exist and knowing exactly which test to request will aid diagnosis as well as fostering a good relationship with your local radiology department.

- High resolution CT of chest ('HRCT') is appropriate where interstitial lung disease or bronchiectasis is suspected and is performed without intravenous contrast.
- CT of thorax with contrast is appropriate in the investigation of lobar collapse, pleural effusion (where diagnostic doubt exists) or where lung cancer or mesothelioma is suspected.
- CT pulmonary angiogram (CTPA) is appropriate in the investigation of suspected PE or pulmonary hypertension.

Ventilation/perfusion (V/Q) scan

This can be requested in the investigation of suspected PE in patients with no evidence of chronic lung disease. It is, however, less specific than CTPA. See Chapter 3 for a discussion of the relative merits of CTPA and V/Q scans in the investigation of suspected PE.

Other investigations

ECG
This can confirm some diagnoses such as heart block and atrial fibrillation. A pulmonary embolism may result in some non-specific ECG changes and these are discussed in detail in Chapter 3. Changes suspicious for pulmonary hypertension include large P waves ('P pulmonale'), right axis deviation, a dominant R wave in lead V1 and right bundle branch block – all of which can be indicative of right ventricular hypertrophy.

Echocardiogram
This is appropriate if cardiac failure has been diagnosed or if valvular heart disease or a cardiomyopathy is suspected. It can also be performed urgently to aid in the diagnosis of a large PE in a shocked patient or to detect acute right ventricular strain.

Peak flow/spirometry
Many patients may be too breathless in an acute situation to perform tests of airway function. In those patients with wheezing (and in particular who are known to have asthma or COPD) and who are able to perform a peak flow or spirometry manoeuvre, a useful baseline measure of airflow obstruction can be gained.

Pleural aspiration
This is often required in the investigation of a unilateral pleural effusion. Fluid should be sent for the following.

- *Protein level.* Classically a pleural fluid protein of >30 g/L is said to indicate an exudate, although lower levels than this can result if the patient is hypoalbuminaemic. Light's criteria may help in distinguishing between a transudate and an exudate.

THINK

What are Light's criteria for pleural fluid analysis?
One of the main elements of diagnostic information to be gained from pleural fluid analysis is whether the fluid is a transudate or an exudate. The simple 'cut-off' of a protein level of 30 g/L may not be reliable and Light's criteria can be used to clarify whether an effusion is likely to be an exudate rather than a transudate by measuring protein and LDH levels in pleural fluid and serum. The fluid is more likely to be an exudate if one or more of the following criteria are met:

- ratio of pleural fluid protein to serum protein >0.5
- ratio of pleural fluid LDH to serum LDH >0.6
- pleural fluid LDH level >66 per cent of normal laboratory serum LDH level.

- *Cytology*. Note that cytology is positive in only 50 per cent of confirmed malignant pleural effusions and false negative results are common. If the fluid is bloodstained on aspiration this is suspicious of malignancy.
- *Microscopy and culture*. Always request this, particularly in the context of pneumonia as an empyema may be present. Request TB culture as well if any risk factors for TB are present.
- *Pleural fluid pH*. In the context of pneumonia with a parapneumonic effusion, a pleural fluid pH < 7.2 is suggestive of infection and should prompt insertion of a chest drain.

Most cases of bilateral pleural effusions are due to cardiac failure or a hypoproteinaemic state (e.g. liver failure, nephrotic syndrome) and aspiration is not usually necessary for diagnostic purposes.

Pleural biopsy
This is the diagnostic investigation of choice in an unexplained unilateral pleural effusion. It is usually performed under

radiological guidance and may need to be performed via thoracoscopy (either under sedation by a specially trained chest physician or by a thoracic surgeon under a general anaesthetic). Diagnoses that can be confirmed by pleural biopsy include:

- metastatic malignancy
- lymphoma
- mesothelioma
- TB of the pleura.

Note that biopsy material should always be sent for TB culture as well as histology if TB is suspected, in order to obtain drug sensitivities that are essential in guiding treatment.

Full lung function tests

Full lung function testing involves measuring spirometry, lung volumes and gas transfer (see **Think** over the page). It is important to note that, although some typical patterns of abnormality exist (emphysema is the best example), full lung function testing cannot usually provide a precise diagnosis. The results of lung function testing should always be interpreted in the light of clinical findings and the results of other (particularly radiological) investigations. Be mindful of the fact that sick, breathless patients often cannot comply with the tests sufficiently to enable a reliable result.

Results will be non-specifically abnormal in any patient with untreated or partially treated cardiac failure or a pleural effusion, for example, and we would argue that there is no diagnostic benefit to be obtained from performing lung function tests in these contexts. However, lung function testing can be particularly helpful in the following situations.

- Interstitial lung disease requires a baseline measure for comparison after treatment and to confirm the typical 'restrictive' pattern of abnormality.
- A raised gas transfer is typical of acute intrapulmonary haemorrhage (the carbon monoxide is taken up by the intra-alveolar blood) and can be used to monitor progress.

- A diagnosis can be confirmed and severity of COPD assessed in a patient recovering from an acute exacerbation.
- Fitness for invasive procedures or surgery can be assessed.
- With unexplained breathlessness, a normal result effectively rules out significant respiratory disease.
- The possibility of respiratory muscle weakness can be assessed.
- Where there is stridor, a flow volume loop can help to localize the possible obstruction to either an intrathoracic or an extrathoracic location as well as quantifying the severity of obstruction.

THINK

What are the limitations of lung function testing?

- Lung function tests provide absolute diagnosis in a minority of conditions (e.g. emphysema).
- The quality of the results is heavily dependent on the technique and expertise of the operator as well as the effort and cooperation of the patient.
- Full lung function testing requires the patient to follow instructions, hold the breath for several seconds (at least) and inspire maximally on several occasions.
- Misleading or unreliable results are often obtained because (a) the patient is too ill to comply with the requirements of the tests; (b) cognitively impaired patients cannot perform the test manoeuvres adequately; or (c) the operator (usually in the case of obtaining simple spirometry) is inadequately trained in the technique.

To obtain the most benefit from lung function testing, obtain the opinion of a respiratory physician.

Exercise oximetry

In cases of diagnostic doubt where a patient reports breathlessness with normal oxygen saturation at rest and no abnormalities on initial laboratory or radiological testing, it is often helpful to walk the patient around (up stairs if possible) with a portable pulse oximeter to monitor oxygen saturation on exertion.

- If the patient becomes visibly breathless with an accompanying fall of more than 4 per cent in oxygen saturation, then a respiratory or cardiac cause is likely and further investigation is warranted.
- If there is no significant drop in oxygen saturation despite observed breathlessness, then significant respiratory disease is unlikely.
- If the patient is overweight and the heart rate rises on fairly minimal exertion with no oxygen desaturation, then the likely cause of exertional breathlessness is lack of fitness.

5 Palpitation

Introduction

The term 'palpitation' means different things to different people. Be prepared for the patient who reports palpitation when merely experiencing an awareness of his or her heartbeats. Alternatively, it may reflect single or multiple extra-systoles: 'My heart just missed a beat, doctor' or 'My heart started thumping and felt as if it was coming out of my chest.' It is important to tease out from these descriptions any suspicion of a genuine tachyarrhythmia (some of which can be life-threatening) from a less serious cause of palpitation.

The differential diagnosis of palpitation will be assisted by the accompanying classification. Various features in the history can help to identify those patients with a significant tachyarrhythmia.

History

What is the rate of palpitation? Ask the patient to reproduce his or her perception of the speed of heartbeat by tapping the back of your hand with their hand. Many patients are capable of giving a fair assessment of heart rate in this way and may be able to differentiate a regular from an irregular heartbeat as well.

● Classification of tachycardias

Sinus tachycardia

If this is confirmed, consider potential causes:
- Substance abuse, including acute alcohol intoxication, caffeine, amphetamines and cocaine
- Drug side-effects, particularly inhaled beta-2 agonists and theophylline preparations for asthma
- Anaemia
- Pregnancy
- Hyperthyroidism
- Anxiety/hyperventilation
- Excessive monosodium glutamate ingestion ('Chinese restaurant syndrome')
- Phaeochromocytoma (very rare)

Supraventricular tachycardias
- Atrial fibrillation
- Atrial flutter
- Atrioventricular nodal re-entrant tachycardia (commonly referred to as SVT or AVRT)

Ventricular tachycardias
- Ventricular tachycardia *per se* almost exclusively (ventricular fibrillation almost always results in sudden death)

Other important aspects of the history are the frequency and duration of episodes of palpitation, and the period over which recurrent episodes have occurred. If recurrent palpitation has been a feature for many years with no adverse outcome then a malignant cause is very unlikely.

Accompanying *chest pain or syncope* is significant and suggestive of a haemodynamically significant dysrhythmia. Presyncope or breathlessness is less discriminative and can be a feature of other conditions such as anxiety or hyperventilation.

Enquire about regular medications or drug use. Antidepressants may indicate a history of anxiety but can also be associated directly with tachyarrhythmia. Beta-2 agonists can cause a rapid heart rate and abnormal rhythms. Is there a history of illicit drug use? What is the consumption of tea, coffee and alcohol?

Enquire about additional symptoms of hyperthyroidism: weight loss, tremor, heat intolerance or irritability. A phaeochromocytoma may present with recurrent episodes of tremor and sweating.

HAZARD

If episodes of palpitation are associated with collapse and/or loss of consciousness, a malignant arrhythmia must be considered likely and urgent investigation is mandatory.

● Examination

Cases with no current palpitation

It is common to be interviewing and examining a patient *between* episodes of palpitation. The examination will then be focused on cardiovascular abnormalities that might relate to cardiac rhythm disturbance.

Evidence of structural heart disease

- Murmurs may point to valvular heart disease.
- A third or a fourth heart sound may indicate myocardial disease, either ischaemic in nature or perhaps secondary to a cardiomyopathy.
- A murmur of left ventricular outflow tract obstruction may be caused by aortic valvular disease, in which case there may be associated changes in the nature of the carotid

pulse and perhaps evidence of left ventricular hypertrophy with a heaving apex beat.

● Examine for evidence of congenital heart disease; atrial septal defect (ASD) is an example.

> **THINK**
>
> The physical signs of an *atrial septal defect* are:
> ● an ejection systolic murmur at the left sternal edge
> ● fixed splitting of the second heart sound
> ● a mid-diastolic murmur over the tricuspid area, which indicates excessive flow through the tricuspid valve (this may be apparent only after exercise).
>
> The vast majority of ASDs are accompanied by right bundle branch block on the ECG.

> **THINK**
>
> Physical signs suggesting haemodynamically significant *aortic outflow tract obstruction* in aortic valve disease are a soft second sound over the aortic area (because of slow closure of the abnormally stiff aortic valve) and a slow-rising carotid pulse.

> **THINK**
>
> The physical signs of *hypertrophic obstructive cardiomyopathy* include evidence of left ventricular hypertrophy, an ejection systolic murmur over the left ventricular outflow tract, possible murmur of mitral regurgitation caused by mechanical tension on the mitral valve as a result of abnormal movement of the hypertrophied interventricular septum, and either a third or a fourth heart sound.

Evidence of associated disease

It is important to lateralize your diagnostic thinking. Is there any clinical evidence for an underlying condition that might precipitate a tachyarrhythmia? Examine for:

- anaemia
- features of thyrotoxicosis (tremor, agitation, thyroid goitre or the eye signs of Grave's disease)
- phaeochromocytoma (acute and markedly elevated blood pressure).

Is there anything to suggest illicit drug abuse – needle marks, unusual behaviour or abnormal neurological findings (e.g. pin-point pupils or diminished corneal reflex, which are both associated with opiate abuse)?

Cases with palpitation present

If rhythm disturbance is present when you are examining the patient this confers a major diagnostic advantage. Under these circumstances it is paramount to recognize and stabilize abnormal haemodynamics and to alleviate any coexisting chest pain. Having ensured this, look for the following:

- **Cannon waves in the neck**. These are characteristic 'flicks' in the jugular venous pressure (JVP) due to intermittent exaggerated atrial waves. They arise when atrial systole occurs against a closed tricuspid valve and are indicative of atrioventricular dissociation. They can be seen with

THINK

In *atrial fibrillation*, the first heart sound is variable in intensity because the irregular nature of the heart rhythm allows variable time for ventricular filling before each systole and the stroke volume has virtual beat-to-beat variability as a result. At rapid heart rates this variability in the first heart sound may be easier to detect than irregularity in rate.

ventricular extra-systoles; but when they are present in association with a sustained tachycardia they are highly suggestive of ventricular tachycardia (VT).

- **Atrial fibrillation**. The pulse is 'irregularly irregular', and this applies to the pulse volume as well as to the pulse rate.

● Investigations

Cases with no current palpitation

If the rhythm disturbance is no longer present, a few investigations will be necessary:

- full blood count, to look for anaemia
- urea and electrolytes – electrolyte abnormalities (particularly abnormal potassium levels) can potentiate myocardial instability
- thyroid function tests
- 12-lead ECG
- chest radiograph, to look for evidence of pulmonary oedema
- echocardiography – important in detecting a structural cardiac abnormality
- 24-hour Holter monitoring.

CLINICAL TIP

If the ECG is normal and there has been no chest pain, there is *no* indication for measuring troponin level.

Cases with palpitation present

If a tachyarrhythmia is still present and is confirmed on ECG, the management plan will depend on the abnormal rhythm shown. Be very careful to obtain ECG evidence as soon as possible. Some common examples follow.

Atrial fibrillation

The clinical finding of an irregularly irregular pulse will be accompanied by irregularity of the QRS complexes on an ECG. The irregularity becomes more difficult to detect with very rapid heart rates, but irregularity of rhythm is usually accompanied by some heterogeneity of the QRS complex morphology.

Atrial flutter

This rhythm is usually not difficult to diagnose on an ECG, because the 'sawtooth' appearance of atrial flutter waves is characteristic. These are not always apparent, though, and there is a simple default position that is largely reliable: namely that any narrow-complex tachycardia of exactly 150/minute (or nearly exactly – see **Think** below) can be assumed to be atrial flutter with 2:1 block, until proved otherwise.

THINK

- The atrial electrical circuit of *atrial flutter* may not manifest as the classical cycle at a frequency of 300/minute. If there is atrial enlargement, the circuit may take longer to complete and the frequency of excitation may fall below 300/minute. If this happens it will be reflected in the ventricular rate according to the existing degree of atrioventricular (a-v) block. For example, in the most common situation of 2:1 block, the observed ventricular rate may be 145/minute and not exactly 150.
- The degree of a-v block may vary (e.g. from 2:1 to 3:1 to 4:1). If this happens, pulse rate and the QRS complexes on an ECG will be irregular as well – so much so that differentiation from atrial fibrillation becomes difficult.

Broad-complex tachycardia

Broad-complex tachycardia (BCT) is defined as a tachycardia with QRS complexes longer than 120 ms in duration (i.e. more than three small squares at the standard ECG speed of 25 mm/s).

In most cases, the differential diagnosis of BCT lies between supraventricular tachycardia with aberrant conduction and ventricular tachycardia. However, it is important to consider the less frequent, but very important, possibility of a tachycardia in association with an accessory pathway. The classical example is the Wolff–Parkinson–White syndrome. There are vitally important therapeutic implications for recognizing this relatively small group of patients, because many drugs that may be used for supraventricular tachycardia are contraindicated in the presence of an accessory pathway.

The salient points in differentiating ventricular tachycardia (VT) from supraventricular tachycardia (SVT) with aberrant conduction are as follows.

- The default position should be to consider VT as the culprit until proved otherwise. It is healthier to assume this, more life-threatening, electrical diagnosis.
- Always look at the patient before spending time analysing the ECG in depth. The patient's clinical condition may demand immediate treatment rather than esoteric discrimination between SVT and VT. The collapsed, hypotensive patient will require immediate cardioversion regardless of the exact nature of his or her dysrhythmia.
- SVT cannot be differentiated from VT on the basis of the patient's clinical condition. VT can be very well tolerated clinically for some time; in contrast, SVT at even relatively modest rates can be poorly tolerated, especially if it arises on the background of structural heart disease.
- If there is a previous history of ischaemic heart disease – and especially one of myocardial infarction – then the

adage 'BCT = VT = cardioversion' has much to commend it. The approach certainly has strong statistical support.

- It is mandatory to examine old case records. Have there been episodes of tachyarrhythmia in the past and, if so, what was the diagnosis? Is there documented evidence of structural heart problems – valvular disease or cardiomyopathy perhaps? Have there been any episodes of heart failure or documentation of ischaemic heart disease? Is there evidence of an electrical problem, such as previous episodes of re-entrant atrioventricular nodal tachycardia, or of an accessory pathway as in Wolff–Parkinson–White or the Lown–Ganong–Levine syndromes?

CLINICAL TIP

Above all else, if the patient has a normal blood pressure, has no chest pain and is not peripherally shut down, you have time to think about preferred therapy. If any of the adverse situations apply, you do not have time and the default management pathway of electrical cardioversion is almost certainly indicated.

HAZARD

Note the importance of implying a 'default' diagnosis of VT rather than SVT.

- In BCT, the default diagnosis is VT rather than SVT.
- Wrongly diagnosing SVT is potentially dangerous. Administration of verapamil in VT, for example, is likely to cause severe and prolonged hypotension or even cardiac arrest.
- Attempts to correct VT, on the other hand, are unlikely to cause further compromise in the patient with SVT.

Electrocardiograph interpretation in BCT

In most cases, broad-complex tachycardia is either SVT with aberrant conduction or VT, and many ECG criteria have been advocated as being helpful in differentiating the two. A number of these are esoteric and difficult to remember.

On the other hand, a diagnosis of VT (remember this is the safer default position) can be made in most instances by asking just a few basic questions on the ECG trace, as follows.

Width of the QRS complex

The wider the QRS complex, the more likely it is to originate from a ventricular focus (Table 5.1).

Table 5.1 Predictive value of QRS complex width in diagnosing ventricular tachycardia

QRS width in seconds	Percentage of cases of VT
Up to 0.12	14
>0.12, up to 0.14	43
>0.14, up to 0.16	100
>0.16, up to 0.18	100
>0.18	100

Atrioventricular dissociation

This is a reliable indicator of VT. Put simply, if P waves can be seen 'marching in and out' of the QRS complexes, this is highly suggestive of VT. An important point is that the opposite is *not* true: atrial and ventricular electrical activity can be associated in VT, particularly if there is retrograde conduction through the a-v node.

Concordance

So-called 'concordance' is present on the ECG if the QRS complexes have the same morphology across the chest leads. The polarization may be all positive (positive concordance) or all negative (negative concordance), and both negative and positive types are reliable indicators of VT.

Capture beats and fusion beats

These are useful pointers to VT.

- A capture beat is a relatively normal QRS complex surrounded by wide complexes. It represents the triggering of ventricular depolarization by the regular atrial activity continuing between abnormal ventricular complexes.
- A fusion beat arises when a capture beat simultaneously depolarizes the ventricles with discharge from the abnormal ventricular focus. This leads to a wide, bizarre complex differing from the QRS complexes surrounding it.

Both phenomena are rare occurrences, but their presence usually secures the diagnosis of VT. (They have been reported rarely in the Wolff–Parkinson–White syndrome and in SVT with bundle branch block.)

Use of adenosine

Adenosine can be used as a diagnostic aid in differentiating VT from SVT, but a few points should be emphasized.

- The drug is a purine nucleoside and is highly effective at completely and transiently blocking the a-v node.

> **⚡ HAZARD**
>
> Adenosine is contraindicated in asthmatics. Also, its use is hazardous if dipyridamole is being taken, because the effects of adenosine are potentiated by this drug.

- Adenosine is very effective in terminating a-v nodal re-entrant tachycardia. It is also useful as a diagnostic tool in uncovering atrial flutter (and perhaps atrial fibrillation) when the ventricular rate is very fast and the underlying rhythm is difficult to determine.
- Adenosine can be used in the haemodynamically stable patient in whom it is impossible to differentiate between

SVT and VT. If it is successful in returning the patient to sinus rhythm, SVT with aberrant conduction is effectively confirmed.

Administer the drug in boluses of 6 mg, and then 12 mg in succession for effect and each followed by a rapid flush. Warn the patient that they may feel awful but only for a few seconds. Larger doses can be given but only under experienced supervision.

Summary

- If the episode of palpitation has ceased, there are some historical and examination findings that are of diagnostic use in determining the cause. In particular, loss of consciousness, chest pain or anything that suggests associated abnormal haemodynamics demands investigation of a potentially malignant arrhythmia.
- If the abnormal rhythm is still present when the patient is seen, then ECG interpretation is fundamental in making the diagnosis. However, the patient's clinical condition is paramount, so correction of abnormal haemodynamics will take priority over detailed diagnosis of the rhythm disturbance.

6 Syncope

● Introduction

Syncope is a cause of temporary loss of consciousness. It has a relatively sudden onset, is self-terminating, and the loss of consciousness is brief, lasting only minutes in most cases. The fundamental cause is a temporary, global interruption of cerebral perfusion.

A rough guide to prevalence of this condition is provided by statistics suggesting that syncope is responsible for 1–3 per cent of emergency department attendances and for 1–6 per cent of hospital admissions.

Before discussing the differential diagnosis it is worth considering that a history of syncope can be difficult to differentiate from a seizure, particularly if no eye-witness account is available. A classical presentation with a witnessed tonic–clonic seizure will present no diagnostic challenge in differentiating a seizure from a syncopal episode; but things are not always as straightforward as this and difficulties are compounded by an incomplete history of the acute event from the patient who will have been unconscious at the time. For these reasons we suggest a simple checklist as a useful starting point in deciding whether the loss of consciousness was truly syncopal, and in particular as an aid to excluding a seizure. *The following features suggest a seizure*:

- bleeding tongue or lip, perhaps noticed on waking
- urinary incontinence

● Classification of syncope

Structural cardiac or cardiopulmonary disease
- Valvular heart disease
- Acute myocardial infarction or ischaemia
- Aortic dissection
- Obstructive cardiomyopathy (uncommon)
- Atrial myxoma (rare)
- Constrictive pericarditis (rare)

Cardiac arrhythmias as a primary cause
- Sinus node dysfunction
- Atrioventricular conduction disease
- Paroxysmal supraventricular and ventricular arrhythmias
- Inherited syndromes predisposing to malignant arrhythmias (long QT and short QT syndromes, Brugada syndrome)
- Implanted cardiac device malfunction
- Drug-induced arrhythmias

Severe pulmonary hypertension
- Acute, due to massive or submassive pulmonary embolism
- Chronic (uncommon), due to primary pulmonary hypertension or chronic thromboembolic pulmonary hypertension, for example

Neurally mediated (reflex)
Those caused by an increase in vagal or parasympathetic tone:
- Vasovagal – the classical 'faint'
- Carotid sinus syncope
- Situational syncope, for example following injections or blood tests in subjects prone to syncope, or on receiving bad news

Orthostatic 'postural' hypotension

- Autonomic nervous system disease due, for example, to diabetes mellitus or Parkinson's disease
- Drug- and alcohol-induced due, for example, to antihypertensives
- Hypovolaemia (blood loss, diarrhoea and vomiting etc.)

Cerebrovascular

- Vascular 'steal' syndromes

- unusual behaviour or unusual olfactory or other sensations before the attack
- other features suggestive of an aura
- post-ictal confusion
- abnormal movements during the episode.

In contrast, the *following suggest a syncopal episode*:

- presyncopal symptoms such as light-headedness or feeling faint
- loss of consciousness in association with prolonged standing or with postural change
- associated sweating.

Having established that the patient is presenting with syncope, the subsequent history and examination should be focused on the potential differential diagnosis. The classification presented here is modified from the European Society of Cardiology guidelines and provides a practical approach to diagnosis based on categorizing the various causes into sub-groups – *this should guide your history and examination*. A few other points are worth making:

- The patient will be unable to give a complete history and eye-witness accounts of the acute event are invaluable.
- Thorough investigation of the previous medical history, drug history and family history are also vital.

- A crucial aspect of your clinical evaluation is to arrive at an assessment of risk for immediate mortality and for potential injury to the patient and others. An obvious example is the risk that would accrue if an episode were to occur when driving. *A guide to risk stratification is provided later in this chapter.*

History

Cardiac syncope

- Is there a history of structural heart disease? Clinical questioning can be guided by the accompanying classification.
- Was the episode associated with exertion? This is very important for 'risk stratification' because several potentially fatal causes present in this way. They include:
  - critical coronary artery disease
  - congenital coronary artery anomaly
  - severe left ventricular outflow tract obstruction (aortic stenosis or hypertrophic obstructive cardiomyopathy)
  - high-grade atrioventricular block
  - catecholamine-triggered ventricular arrhythmias (the long Q–T syndrome is the classical example because catecholamines of exercise potentiate this inherited abnormality of calcium channels in heart muscle cells)
  - severe pulmonary hypertension.
- Syncope occurring when supine is a serious feature and is commonly associated with a cardiac cause, particularly an arrhythmia.
- Was there a history of palpitation preceding the episode?
- Are negatively inotropic or chronotropic drugs being prescribed, such as beta-blockers or verapamil?
- Is there a family history of sudden death? While this may be indicative of familial ischaemic heart disease, it may also signal one of a variety of inherited conditions that can first present as syncope. Long and short Q–T syndromes,

arrhythmogenic right ventricular dysplasia (ARVD) and Brugada syndrome are examples.

- Is there an implantable cardiac device? This may be faulty.
- Are there any risk factors for a pulmonary embolism (PE)? See Chapter 3 p. 36 for a full description of risk factors for PE.

Postural hypotension

- Is there an obvious association with postural change? See the **Clinical tip** below).
- Is there an association with relevant drug administration, or has a new prescription for antihypertensives or other potentially culpable drug types been administered?
- Prolonged standing (especially with older patients and especially if it is hot) is a suggestive feature.
- Is there a history of autonomic nervous system disease or a condition predisposing to it? Diabetes, Parkinson's disease and the Shy–Drager syndrome are examples.

CLINICAL TIP

A very rare cause of postural syncope is an *atrial myxoma*. A young patient with this condition presented with recurrent episodes of loss of consciousness when sitting up (on several occasions when being examined by medical staff!). The left atrial myxoma shifted position with the postural change to block the mitral valve and therefore left ventricular inflow. The obstruction was immediately corrected as the patient collapsed and became supine.

Neurally mediated ('reflex') syncope

Consider this as a possible cause if there is:

- no evidence of cardiac disease
- a long history of recurrent syncope
- a relationship with pain, an emotive event, or perhaps an unexpected sight, sound or smell

- prolonged standing in crowded, hot places
- accompanying nausea, vomiting or blurring of vision
- syncope while eating or immediately afterwards
- an association with head rotation (causing pressure on the carotid sinus) – the history may reveal syncope when shaving, when in church, or if wearing a tight collar.

Cerebrovascular 'steal' syndromes

These are uncommon and are caused by partial arterial obstruction secondary to atherosclerosis. The classic example is syncope associated with arm exercise – the 'subclavian steal syndrome'.

CLINICAL TIP

Some patients do not fit convincingly into any of the above groups of conditions. It is then safer to assume that either cardiac syncope or perhaps pulmonary embolism may be responsible – and investigate accordingly.

● Examination

Cardiovascular exam

Examine for:

- irregular and/or rapid heart rate
- hypotension
- postural hypotension (perform lying and sitting or standing blood pressure measurements)
- paradoxical pulse and blood pressure, indicative of pericardial constriction or effusion causing cardiac tamponade
- postural changes in heart rate
- structural heart disease (see **Think** below)
- heart failure.

THINK

What structural heart disease might be relevant?

- Murmurs will point to valvular problems.
- A third heart sound or gallop rhythm suggests myocardial disease, which may be ischaemic or due to a cardiomyopathy.
- A fourth heart sound may accompany obstructive cardiomyopathy, aortic stenosis or heart failure.
- The slow-rising carotid pulse of aortic stenosis is characteristic and is often accompanied by a soft aortic second sound (the stiff and diseased aortic valve closes slowly and quietly).
- The collapsing pulse of aortic regurgitation and the (now rare) bisferiens pulse of mixed aortic valve disease are similarly unmistakeable.
- Differences in blood pressure in each arm. A discrepancy may indicate aortic dissection.

Look too for signs of *pulmonary hypertension*: a raised jugular venous pressure, loud pulmonary second sound and right ventricular hypertrophy. These changes may be acute due to pulmonary embolism or indicative of chronic pulmonary hypertension (when ankle swelling may also be a feature).

HAZARD

Carotid sinus massage may produce the bradycardia diagnostic of carotid sinus hypersensitivity. Perform this with caution as it may precipitate a syncopal episode.

Neurological examination

A careful and comprehensive neurological examination is important. Look for evidence of involuntary movements, abnormal tone and bradykinesia suggestive of Parkinson's disease.

General examination

Dehydration, debility and anaemia are predisposing features for syncopal events.

● Investigations

Some common causes of syncope have no confirmatory diagnostic tests; examples are vasovagal episodes, carotid sinus sensitivity and postural hypotension. These diagnoses are dependent on a good history and suggestive features on examination. Specialist referral to a cardiologist will usually be indicated if cardiac syncope is suspected. Investigations that should be considered include the following.

- *Full blood count*. Look for anaemia or evidence of infection.
- *Urea and electrolytes*. Look for electrolyte abnormalities or evidence of dehydration.
- *Cardiac troponin*. If elevated, this can indicate cardiac ischaemia or pulmonary embolism.
- *ECG*. This provides vital information and studies have shown that the majority of diagnoses of syncope are made with careful clinical assessment complemented by a 12-lead ECG. Table 6.1 summarizes the specific ECG features to look for, and Table 6.2 lists the ECG findings that are considered to be diagnostic of an arrhythmia-associated syncope.
- *Echocardiography*. This is the investigation of choice to confirm suspected valvular lesions, cardiomyopathy, pulmonary hypertension or other structural cardiac disease. Other imaging techniques (e.g. cardiac MRI) may be necessary to investigate unusual structural abnormalities and cardiomyopathy.
- *CT pulmonary angiography*. Is PE suspected?
- *Coronary angiography*. This may be indicated if ischaemic heart disease is suspected.
- *24-hour Holter monitoring*. This may be indicated to investigate for potential arrhythmia.

- *Specialist cardiology services*. These may also undertake implantable loop recording of cardiac events over a longer period of time, and can check the function of any implanted cardiac devices (e.g. pacemakers).
- *Tilt-table testing*. This may be indicated if autonomic dysfunction is suspected. It will require specialist assessment and referral.

Table 6.1 ECG abnormalities to look for in the syncopal patient

Bifascicular block: left bundle branch block or right bundle branch block with either left anterior or left posterior fascicular block
Prolonged QRS interval (>120 ms)
Evidence of pulmonary embolism: sinus tachycardia, non-specific ST segment abnormalities. The often quoted S wave in lead 1, Q wave in lead 3 and inverted T wave in lead 3 indicate acute life-threatening right ventricular strain
Mobitz 1 second-degree heart block (Wenckebach phenomenon)
Sinus node disease (sinus bradycardia <50 beats/min, sinoatrial block, spontaneous sinus arrest with duration of >3 s)
Evidence of pre-excitation (e.g. the delta wave of Wolff–Parkinson–White or the short PR interval of Lown–Ganong–Levine syndrome)
Prolonged QT interval (defined as a QTc of >440 ms)
Abnormal ST segments in leads V1–V3, suggestive of Brugada syndrome
T-wave inversion in right precordial leads and perhaps accompanying epsilon waves of ARVD
Changes of myocardial infarction or ischaemia

ARVD, arrhythmogenic right ventricular dysplasia

Table 6.2 Diagnostic ECG changes for an arrhythmia-associated syncope

Sinus bradycardia <40 beats/min
Repetitive sinoatrial block or sinus arrest of >3 s
Mobitz 2 second-degree heart block
Third-degree heart block
Alternating left and right bundle branch block
Rapid supraventricular tachycardia
Ventricular tachycardia
Pacemaker malfunction

● Risk stratification of the syncopal patient

As mentioned at the start of this chapter, a primary aim of the assessment of the patient with syncope is to attempt to quantify the degree of individual risk based on clinical criteria. This has been the focus of considerable research and several prognostic markers identify patients at risk. We end this chapter with a discussion of risk stratification in order to emphasize those patients who require hospital investigation of their symptoms.

Highest mortality risk indicating the need for in-hospital investigation

This category is associated with the following:

- acute myocardial ischaemia or infarction
- aortic dissection
- congestive heart failure
- structural heart disease including valvular pathology, pulmonary hypertension and pericardial disease
- ECG changes including high-degree atrioventricular block, cardiac rhythm pauses of more than 2–3 s, pre-excitation syndromes, suspected ARVD, and inherited syndromes associated with malignant arrhythmia (Q–T interval abnormalities and Brugada syndromes).
- syncope during exercise
- syncope resulting in motor vehicle accidents or personal injury
- a family history of sudden death
- the presence of an implanted cardiac device.

Low mortality risk

This category is associated with the following:

- no evidence of structural heart disease
- a normal baseline ECG.

Although the immediate threat to life is low in this group, the risk of injury due to recurrent falls has to be considered. There are also implications for particular occupations (handling machinery, working at height etc.), fitness to drive, and safety of air travel. The decision to admit to hospital for investigations will always be an individual one and dictated by a number of considerations.

7 Seizures

Introduction

The occurrence of a seizure (or 'fit') is a common reason for presentation at emergency departments. Approximately 5 per cent of people will experience a seizure at some point during their life and most will not have epilepsy. Given a sufficient trigger, any of us could experience a seizure as we all have a 'seizure threshold'. The emphasis in this chapter is on the investigation of causes of seizures in a hospital emergency department rather than a detailed discussion of the diagnosis of epilepsy, which often requires non-urgent specialist input.

The first challenge is to identify whether the abnormal movement reported is actually a seizure, as not all abnormal movement constitutes seizure activity. Getting the diagnosis of a seizure correct is important for several reasons, not least because having a seizure diagnosed usually leads to restrictions on driving and may adversely affect employment and personal insurance prospects. There are some features in the history and examination that help to decide whether the event described is a true seizure or not.

● Classification of seizures

Common causes

- Epilepsy – seizures can occur despite adequate treatment in epileptic patients, or be triggered by the following:
  - Poor compliance with treatment, or recent change in treatment
  - Intercurrent illness, particularly infection
  - Alcohol (excess or withdrawal)
  - Fatigue
  - Hypoglycaemia (missed meals)
- Alcohol – both alcohol excess and withdrawal can lead to seizures
- Hypoglycaemia
- Electrolyte disturbance – usually profound in order to cause seizures:
  - Hyponatraemia: the serum sodium is usually <115 mmol/L
  - Hypocalcaemia: usually <1.5 mmol/L
  - Hypomagnesaemia – usually occurs in conjunction with hypocalcaemia and the hypocalcaemia will be difficult to correct if the serum magnesium is not corrected at the same time
  - Uraemia – usually >50 mmol/L
- Recreational drug use – cocaine, amphetamines and ecstasy are examples
- Cerebrovascular disease – acute stroke or chronic cerebrovascular disease
- Head injury
- Acute intracranial haemorrhage:
  - Subarachnoid haemorrhage
  - Primary intracerebral haemorrhage
  - Extradural haemorrhage
  - Subdural haemorrhage

- Acute cerebral hypoperfusion – usually follows sudden loss of cardiac output; the most common causes are cardiological and include life-threatening brady- and tachyarrhythmias
- Acute hypoxaemia from any cause

Less common causes of seizures

- Intracerebral space-occupying lesions – examples include primary and secondary brain tumours and cerebral abscess
- Intracranial infection – such as encephalitis and meningitis
- Cerebral vasculitis
- Hyperthermia – a core body temperature of >40.5°C caused by:
  - Heat stroke during very hot weather (Patients vulnerable to heat stroke are those taking antipsychotic medication, elderly patients with chronic medical conditions such as cardiac failure and subjects undertaking extreme exercise such as soldiers on military manoeuvres and marathon runners)
  - Ecstasy ingestion
  - Neuroleptic malignant syndrome (a rare idiosyncratic reaction to neuroleptic medication, it comprises muscle rigidity, hyperthermia and impaired consciousness. Gross elevation of serum creatine phosphokinase (CK) is a feature.)
  - Malignant hyperthermia – a rare inherited reaction to some anaesthetic agents
- Hypertensive encephalopathy (briefly described in the chapter on acute headache)
- Eclampsia – now an uncommon cause of seizures in countries with well-developed antenatal services
- *Plasmodium falciparum* malaria

THINK

What features of the history and examination increase the likelihood of a true seizure rather than non-seizure activity?

- Tongue biting, usually of the side of the tongue, is very suggestive of a seizure.
- After a generalized grand mal seizure most patients will exhibit a post-ictal phase lasting up to several hours during which they are drowsy, confused or deeply asleep.
- Incontinence is often quoted as a feature but is less reliable and not specific to seizures.
- A good eye-witness account with a clear description of the event is invaluable and goes a long way to confirming whether or not the episode described was a seizure.

The 'language' of seizures

Seizures are classified in a number of different ways and a reliable eye-witness account is required to classify an event accurately. A simplified version of the international classification of seizures is as follows.

Generalized seizures

These involve all of the cerebral cortex, and seizure activity therefore involves the whole body. Consciousness is always impaired. Generalized seizures can be further classified as follows:

- *convulsive* – most commonly a tonic–clonic 'grand mal' seizure (this is the type of seizure that most often precipitates a presentation to emergency medical services)
- *non-convulsive* – for example, absence seizures known classically as 'petit mal'.

Note also that some generalized seizures may be tonic only, without a clonic phase. Patients will appear to be stiff and unresponsive, with rigid muscles. This is often not recognized by inexperienced staff as a seizure.

Partial seizures

These begin in a focal part of the cerebral cortex, so the seizure motor activity begins in one area (such as the face or arm). It may then become generalized or remain focal. Partial seizures are subclassified as:

- *simple* – meaning there is no impairment of consciousness
- *complex* – meaning there is an impaired conscious level.

Status epilepticus

This is a term referring to prolonged seizures. It is a medical emergency that requires immediate treatment.

THINK

What is status epilepticus?
Seizures which continue unabated or recur quickly over a period of more than 30 minutes. The most common manifestation is of prolonged grand mal seizure activity in a known epileptic. When occurring *de novo* in a non-epileptic patient, there is a high chance of the presence of serious intracranial pathology such as infection or a space-occupying lesion. Status epilepticus can also occur in non-convulsive forms of seizures which can lead to diagnostic difficulty: patients may then present with prolonged confusion and altered consciousness, often misinterpreted as delirium.
In non-convulsive status epilepticus there may be only very subtle motor signs of seizure activity such as

fluttering of the eyelids, nystagmoid movements of the eyes or akathisia (odd involuntary movements of the tongue or lower jaw).

HAZARD

Status epilepticus is a medical emergency as prolonged seizures can lead to permanent brain damage. It must be treated immediately with intravenous antiepileptic agents to terminate seizure activity before further investigations are undertaken.

Conditions often misinterpreted as seizures

- **Vasovagal episode**. Some patients with a severe vasovagal episode will exhibit twitching of the limbs after fainting. This can be mistaken easily for seizure activity but true tonic–clonic motor activity is absent. A good history should indicate the likely diagnosis of a vasovagal episode. Patients usually feel 'faint' for some minutes beforehand and there are often precipitating factors such as prolonged standing, hot weather or dehydration.

- **Pseudoseizures**. Some patients will present to emergency departments with feigned generalized seizures. The underlying psychological reasons for this are usually complex and beyond the scope of this text. Pseudoseizures are also well documented in epileptic patients. Differentiating a pseudoseizure from a genuine seizure can be difficult, but there are a few clues (see **Think** below).

- **Myoclonus**. Myoclonus is brief repetitive muscle twitches or jerks. There are many potential causes (including much overlap with causes of seizures).

In particular, patients with any form of brain damage may exhibit myoclonus and this is easily mistaken for seizure activity.

THINK

What features help to distinguish a pseudoseizure from a genuine seizure?
Common features of a pseudoseizure include eyes that are tightly shut, pelvic thrusting, thrashing movements of the limbs, duration longer than two minutes, and absence of post-ictal drowsiness. After the event a serum prolactin level may help: it is usually raised after a true seizure and not raised by a pseudoseizure.

● History

Most patients who have just experienced a seizure will be unable to give a history for some hours while they are post-ictal. At best you may be able to interview a witness about the acute episode and will have to return when the patient has regained consciousness (and after initial investigations) to complete the clerking. An eye-witness account of the episode is in any case the only description you will be able to obtain to confirm a generalized seizure as the patient will have had impaired consciousness at the time. You may be in a situation where no background history is available at all and you will need to proceed immediately to investigations. If possible, seek answers to the following:

- *Is the patient known to be epileptic?* If so, ask about:
  – compliance with medication
  – recent changes to medication
  – recent illness
  – alcohol intake
  – lifestyle factors such as sleep deprivation and haphazard mealtimes.

- *Ask all patients about alcohol intake*, both recent and habitual. Acute alcohol intoxication and withdrawal from alcohol in habitual heavy drinkers can both precipitate seizures.
- *Is the patient diabetic?* Hypoglycaemia could be a possible cause of the seizure.
- *Is there a history of recreational drug use?* Note that many patients (and witnesses) may deny this even if it has been a factor.
- *Has the patient sustained a head injury in the last few days?* A seizure in this context raises the possibility of an extradural haemorrhage. This is a life-threatening medical emergency requiring immediate investigation with a CT scan of the head (see Chapter 10).
- *Are there any symptoms of current illness?* A respiratory tract infection may cause hypoxia, or diarrhoea/vomiting may result in electrolyte imbalance.
- *Is there a drug history?* Some drugs (e.g. diuretics) can lead to electrolyte imbalance. Others (e.g. neuroleptics) can be rare causes of seizures via mechanisms listed above. If no other background history is available, seek evidence of prescribed medication from relatives and the general practitioner.
- *What is the past medical history?* In the context of a seizure, a history of previous malignancy with a propensity to metastasize to the brain may be significant. Common examples are lung and breast cancer and malignant melanoma.
- *Has there been recent foreign travel?* Ask this with the possibility of malaria in mind, particularly if the patient is febrile.
- *If the patient is of child-bearing age, could she be pregnant?* Ask this with two things in mind: the possibility (albeit rare in industrialized countries) of eclampsia, and the implications it may have for ongoing pharmacological management of epilepsy.

● Examination

For reasons already mentioned, you will often be in a situation of examining a post-ictal patient before being able to obtain a background history. The examination of a drowsy or unconscious patient is challenging as they are unable to comply with normal commands. A lot of information can still be gathered even in these suboptimal circumstances. Bearing in mind the causes of seizures, look in particular for the following.

General examination

- *'MedicAlert' bracelet*. This might give you valuable information such as whether the patient is epileptic or diabetic.
- *Pulse rate*. Look for an arrhythmia.
- *Sepsis*. Is the patient febrile or hypotensive? Is the respiratory rate raised, and are there any rashes? The presence of signs of sepsis raises the possibility that the seizure may have been caused by:
  - meningitis or encephalitis (see chapter 10 for a fuller description of the causes of intracranial infection)
  - pneumonia (leading to hypoxia)
  - malaria.

CLINICAL TIP

Bear in mind that a transient ('single spike') moderate rise in temperature is common after a seizure because of repetitive muscle contraction. If you suspect sepsis, then start treatment with intravenous broad-spectrum antibiotics as delay in treating bacterial meningitis can prove fatal. If the patient has a core temperature of 40°C or above, consider hyperthermia as the primary diagnosis. In addition to empirical antibiotic treatment, the patient must be cooled promptly as the cause is sought.

- *Alcoholic foetor.* This may indicate acute intoxication as the cause.
- *Stigmata of chronic liver disease.* Spider naevi, palmar erythema, leuconychia, ascites, bruising and bleeding into the skin, poor nutrition and muscle wasting are all signs of chronic alcohol abuse and raise the possibility of seizures due to alcohol withdrawal.
- *Signs of intravenous drug abuse.* Look for needle track marks, for instance.
- *Scalp lacerations.* These could suggest a recent head injury.
- *Blood pressure.* If there is marked hypertension (e.g. diastolic >140 mmHg), this may indicate hypertensive encephalopathy which is the most serious manifestation of malignant hypertension. Other features of malignant hypertension include renal failure and papilloedema.

Neurological examination

Perform as complete a neurological examination as possible. In a drowsy or semi-conscious patient you may only be able to document the level of consciousness (e.g. using the Glasgow Coma Scale), the presence of spontaneous limb movement, pupillary reflexes, limb tone and reflexes. In addition you should be able to perform adequate fundoscopy to look for papilloedema. Good patient cooperation is required, however, for accurate documentation of power, sensation, coordination and cranial nerve examination. Obvious asymmetry in pupil size, limb tone, reflexes or movement may point towards significant intracranial pathology such as a stroke, space-occupying lesion or intracranial bleeding.

● Investigations

A number of simple bedside and laboratory tests should be performed as soon as possible in any patient who has had a seizure or who is in status epilepticus.

Bedside and laboratory tests

- *Bedside blood glucose measurement from a fingerprick test.* A patient who is hypoglycaemic must be treated immediately with intravenous dextrose.
- *Pulse oximetry*, looking for hypoxaemia. If the patient is hypoxaemic then administer oxygen immediately and perform arterial blood gas analysis to look for acid–base disturbance and/or evidence of respiratory failure.
- *Blood biochemistry*:
  - serum urea and electrolytes (look in particular at the sodium and urea levels in the context of a seizure)
  - serum calcium
  - random blood glucose (in addition to the fingerprick test listed above)
  - liver function tests (for evidence of chronic liver disease)
  - serum magnesium if hypocalcaemia is present.
- *Full blood count.* If the patient is febrile, check the white cell and neutrophil counts.
- *Blood cultures.* Obtain these in any febrile patient who has had a seizure.
- *Urine dipstick and MSU*, for culture in any febrile patient.
- *ECG.* Perform this after seizure activity has ceased, looking for evidence of an arrhythmia. During a seizure it will not be possible to obtain an ECG trace owing to muscle activity.

Special cases

- In all women of child-bearing age, do a pregnancy test: blood or urine human chorionic gonadotrophin (HCG) levels.
- In a febrile patient with a recent history of travel to a malaria endemic area, send several blood samples for a thick film to look for malarial parasites. A single negative result does not exclude malaria.

Radiological investigations

The main radiological test for consideration is CT of the head. In a known epileptic this is usually not necessary unless there is something new or unusual about the pattern of the seizure. A CT scan is otherwise indicated in the following circumstances:

- a 'first seizure' in an adult patient
- recent head injury
- the presence of focal neurology, raising the possibility of a space-occupying lesion, stroke or intracranial bleed
- fever.

CLINICAL TIP

Fever may indicate intracranial infection such as meningitis or encephalitis. In this circumstance it is best practice to perform a CT scan of the head before attempting a diagnostic lumbar puncture in order to assess the potential risk of cerebral herniation or 'coning'. See Chapter 10 for a fuller discussion.

A CT scan of the head will be sufficient to make a diagnosis in most cases of intracranial bleeding and space-occupying lesion. It is often most helpful in ruling out these potential causes of a seizure.

In a febrile, septic or hypoxaemic patient, a chest x-ray (CXR) is also indicated to look for a cause. Bear in mind that a supine CXR in a semi-conscious or unconscious patient is often of very poor quality and accurate interpretation of films in this context is challenging. You may need to repeat the CXR under better circumstances once the patient has regained consciousness.

Other tests

- *Lumbar puncture*. Obtain cerebrospinal fluid for examination (a detailed description of this process can be found in Chapter 10). In the context of a seizure, a lumbar puncture should be performed only after a CT of the head and if it is deemed safe to proceed – the decision regarding this should be made at a senior level. The indications for a lumbar puncture are:
  - suspected meningitis
  - suspected encephalitis
  - strong clinical suspicion of subarachnoid haemorrhage (SAH) with a normal CT of the head, particularly if the patient has presented more than 24 hours after the onset of symptoms (see Chapter 10 for a fuller discussion of SAH).
- *Electroencephalography*. This should be undertaken after specialist advice from a neurologist. Interpreting the results is a specialized skill. An EEG can provide a diagnosis in some forms of epilepsy and encephalitis (e.g. herpes simplex encephalitis). Performing an EEG immediately after a seizure is not usually helpful in identifying the cause of a seizure.

⚡ HAZARD

After diagnosing a seizure from any cause you must ascertain whether the patient has a current driving licence. Familiarize yourself with the regulations in force where you practise, and advise current drivers appropriately regarding initial driving restrictions after a seizure. The rules vary, but an initial 6- to12-month period of suspension of a driving licence is usual after a single seizure. Your responsibility is to inform the patient of any initial restriction and advise him or her to contact the relevant licensing authority. It is not usually the responsibility of the doctor to contact the licensing authority.

HAZARD

Do not diagnose epilepsy after a single seizure in a young adult if you have not found an identifiable cause. A diagnosis of epilepsy should be made by a specialist after appropriate consideration and investigation, as it can have profound effects on employment and lifestyle.

8 Dizziness

● Introduction

Dizziness is an imprecise term used to describe a variety of unpleasant sensations of imbalance or altered orientation in space. Normal balance relies on intact visual, vestibular and proprioceptive sensation and, in health, these sensory modalities combine to provide an accurate perception of one's surroundings. Symptoms of dizziness or imbalance can accrue if one is exposed to an unrecognized combination of sensory inputs triggered by exposure to odd visual stimuli. Flickering images on a TV screen or fast-moving traffic are examples of this phenomenon. In addition, symptoms are associated with disease involving visual, vestibular or proprioceptive sensation or a combination of these.

It follows that the actual symptoms experienced will vary according to the nature of the pathology, but the term 'dizziness' is often used generically by patients to describe a variety of sensations of imbalance. Determining what is meant by 'dizziness' in an individual situation is crucial to diagnosis and it is useful to categorize the possibilities as follows.

- **Vertigo**. This is an illusion of movement in relation to the environment. It is most commonly 'rotatory' in nature: 'the room is spinning around me', or perhaps the patient feels that he or she is spinning around the room. Occasionally, the perceived sensations are different; body tilting, swaying and forceful movement (impulsion – 'being pushed in the back') are examples.

● Classification of dizziness

Many **drugs** can cause unspecified 'dizziness'. Common examples include anticonvulsants and proton pump inhibitors.

Vertigo

- Acute labyrinthitis (also known as vestibular neuronitis)
- Benign positional paroxysmal vertigo (BPPV)
- Posterior circulation stroke
- Ménière's disease
- Vertebrobasilar migraine
- Multiple sclerosis
- Anxiety/hyperventilation syndrome
- Brain-stem tumour
- Head injury

Disequilibrium

- Visual impairment
- Peripheral neuropathy
- Dorsal column dysfunction – the classic example is subacute combined degeneration of the cord due to vitamin B_{12} deficiency
- Disease of the vestibular component of the 8th nerve – e.g. compression by a tumour, the direct toxic effect of aminoglycoside antibiotics
- Toxic blood levels of anticonvulsants, barbiturates and alcohol – all capable of impairing brain-stem and cerebellar function

Pre-syncope

This is common in older patients with pre-existing medical conditions. Causes include:
- Ischaemic heart disease
- Valvular heart disease, particularly aortic stenosis
- Antihypertensive therapy

- Anaemia
- Autonomic neuropathy, for example due to diabetes mellitus or Parkinson's disease
- Hypoglycaemia
- Postural hypotension – often drug-induced, particularly by antihypertensives

- **Disequilibrium**. This is a sensation of disordered balance. It is described as static if it is experienced when standing and dynamic if it occurs when walking. 'Unsteadiness' and 'loss of balance' are descriptions commonly used by patients and recurrent falling is a common accompaniment.
- **Presyncope**. This is a sensation of impending loss of consciousness, usually due to an acute reduction in blood pressure or cardiac output. Patients describe 'light-headedness', 'feeling faint' or 'feeling woozy'. Sweating, pallor, nausea and visual symptoms of 'dimming' or 'blurring' are common associations. The causes include many common chronic medical conditions.

THINK

What are the causes of vertigo and disequilibrium?
- *Vertigo* is a false sensation of movement, which is often rotatory, and caused by disease of the vestibular system, the cerebellum or the neurological pathways between these structures.
- *Disequilibrium* is a term for disordered balance and it can accrue from disturbance of any of the sensory systems responsible for normal balance; namely, the visual, proprioceptive and vestibular systems. In disequilibrium, focused clinical assessment of all three sensory modalities is required.

Neuroanatomy

Some knowledge of the anatomy of the systems responsible for normal balance is helpful in understanding the common causes of dizziness and how to differentiate between them.

- The vestibular system in the inner ear detects rotational and linear acceleration. It combines with visual and proprioceptive sensory input to maintain body orientation in space. Abnormal function of the vestibular system results in vertigo.
- Abnormal proprioception (one of the causes being disease of the dorsal columns) results in unsteadiness and this is compounded severely if vision is also abnormal. This is the basis of Romberg's test, which is described later. A patient with both abnormal proprioception and vision will present with profound unsteadiness and recurrent falls.
- Sensory information from the vestibular system is transmitted by the vestibular division of the 8th cranial nerve. This travels with the cochlear nerve (which carries auditory information) through the petrous temporal bone to the internal auditory meatus. The 8th nerve then traverses the subarachnoid space in the cerebello-pontine angle to synapse in the vestibular nuclei on the floor of the fourth ventricle at the ponto-medullary junction.

The vestibular nuclei subsequently project sensory information to the following systems.

- **Cerebellum**. This is the functional centre for balance and coordination. Ataxia will result if there is disturbed sensory input to this system.
- **Parieto-temporal cortex**. These projections are responsible for the conscious perception of spatial orientation and motion. Disturbance of their sensory inputs will result in vertigo, and this may occur either because of discordant input from the right and left

vestibules or from a conflict between vestibular and other sensory input.

- **Oculomotor nuclei**. These regulate vestibulo-ocular reflexes, which are responsible for maintaining steady gaze. Vestibular nystagmus, which commonly accompanies vertigo, results from a disturbance in this reflex system.
- **Spinal cord**. The vestibulo-spinal tract assists in maintaining posture and balance, explaining why unsteadiness is a common occurrence in vestibular disease.

This simplified anatomical account leads to the traditional distinction between *peripheral vertigo* (arising from the labyrinth or the vestibular nerve) and *central vertigo* (arising from brain-stem or vestibular connections).

THINK

Do symptoms help to differentiate between peripheral and central causes of vertigo?

- A consideration of the neuroanatomy described above explains why accompanying symptomatology aids in classifying vertigo accurately into one of these two basic categories: accompanying deafness supports a peripheral aetiology while other brain-stem symptoms (diplopia, dysarthria, facial numbness, limb weakness etc.) suggest a central cause.
- The nature and direction of the vertigo itself is not infallible in allowing accurate classification although peripheral, rotational vertigo is usually in a 'yaw' plane (horizontal rotation, 'spinning'). Vertigo in other planes, forward and back ('pitch') and side-to-side ('roll'), should raise suspicion of central pathology (Fig. 8.1).

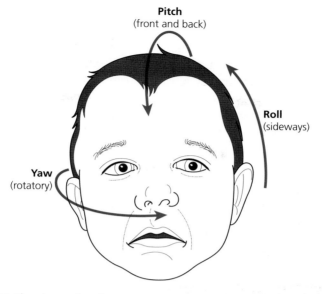

Fig. 8.1 The planes of vertigo

● History

An accurate history will involve direct questioning and, because
analysis of the presenting complaint on its own may not clarify
the diagnosis, it is important to explore other aspects of the
history.

Speed of onset and accompanying systemic upset

Ask whether the onset was sudden or gradual. Sudden onset of vertigo is usually very disabling, being accompanied by nausea and profound vomiting. *Acute labyrinthitis* (also known as vestibular neuronitis) is a classic cause and presents with vertigo, nausea, vomiting, ataxia and nystagmus. Movement aggravates the symptoms and the patient lies still in bed during the acute phase, very wary of exacerbating the unpleasant symptoms. Nystagmus is the only abnormal neurological sign.

Benign paroxysmal positional vertigo (BPPV) tends to occur suddenly, but other features help to differentiate it from acute labyrinthitis (Table 8.1).

Posterior circulation stroke can be responsible for acute vertigo. Although systemic upset may occur in the early stages, nausea and vomiting are usually less severe and tend to be less persistent.

A more *gradual onset* of vertigo is seen in Ménière's disease, vertebrobasilar migraine, brain-stem tumour, demyelination, drug intoxication and anxiety disorders including hyperventilation.

Duration of symptoms

Ask whether this is the first episode or whether there have been repeated episodes over time.

- BPPV is typically episodic with recurrent episodes lasting minutes at most. The typical periodicity involves repeated attacks (sometimes several each day) over a period of a week or two followed by spontaneous resolution of symptoms for a variable period of time, often for months.
- Acute labyrinthitis tends to be severely disabling for 2–5 days and minor symptoms often continue for a few weeks thereafter. During the 'convalescent' phase there can be a positional element to the symptoms and the patient will often walk with his or her head held immobile on their shoulders in an attempt to avoid positional vertigo.

Table 8.1 Differentiating features in some common conditions presenting with vertigo

Condition	Features
Acute labyrinthitis, often called 'vestibular neuronitis' and attributed to an acute viral illness (but with little evidence). May occur in mini-epidemics	Gradual onset, symptoms persist for days or even weeks Episodes may be recurrent/accompanying nausea, vomiting and ataxia, which is often severe Any age group Nystagmus is the only abnormal physical sign
Benign paroxysmal positional vertigo	Sudden onset, brief duration (often only seconds), episodic Clear relation to a particular head position Older age group Positive Dix–Hallpike manoeuvre
Méniére's disease	Gradual onset, symptoms for hours or days, episodic Sensorineural hearing loss
Brain-stem stroke	Sudden onset, symptoms for days or weeks, may be recurrent Nausea and vomiting at outset and tend not to persist Other brain-stem symptoms/signs Older age group Cardiovascular risk factors
Brain-stem tumour	As above, but more gradual onset and with progressive symptoms and signs
Vertebro-basilar migraine	Gradual onset, duration hours to 2 days, often recurrent Associated throbbing headache and/or visual disturbance Often younger patients
Demyelination	Gradual onset, symptoms and signs may persist for weeks, may be recurrent Associated neurological signs Previous neurological symptoms and/or signs suggesting multiple site involvement

Acute labyrinthitis can be recurrent but does not manifest the characteristic periodicity of BPPV.

● Ménière's disease is also recurrent and can be episodic. In this condition, vertigo becomes less marked as hearing loss becomes more pronounced. Each episode of vertigo lasts for hours or days. A history of migraine is common in Ménière's disease.

- Vertigo secondary to demyelination can be monophasic or recurrent, as can that due to posterior circulation stroke or vertebrobasilar migraine. The latter tends to resolve within 24 hours, but stroke and demyelination are responsible for symptoms that can last for weeks.

- Progressive vertigo is typical of brain-stem tumour, other structural brain-stem pathology (e.g. Chiari malformation) and the bilateral vestibular paresis of the elderly.

Posture and other triggering factors

- The classical cause of vertigo related to posture is BPPV, where the symptoms are short-lived and related to changing head position. Attacks typically occur when getting into or out of bed or on rolling from one side to the other. Changes of head position in specific circumstances (e.g. in church) can also precipitate BPPV.

- Acute labyrinthitis can be exacerbated by position during both its acute and convalescent phases. The patient lies still in bed to avoid unpleasant systemic symptoms triggered when the vestibular system is stimulated by movement.

- Postural hypotension can mimic positional vertigo, but here the symptoms occur typically when getting out of bed or with other postural changes. A systolic blood pressure drop of more than 20 mmHg on standing from a supine position supports the diagnosis.

- Walking in the dark can exacerbate vestibular pathology, but dizziness or unsteadiness occurring exclusively in the dark suggests an abnormality of proprioception (e.g. peripheral neuropathy or subacute combined degeneration of the cord).

- The transient increase in intracranial pressure that occurs with defaecation, coughing, sneezing or bending over can worsen vertigo caused by a posterior fossa mass lesion or malformation (e.g. Chiari malformation).

Age

- The differential diagnosis of vertigo in younger patients includes acute labyrinthitis, Ménière's disease, medication (e.g. anticonvulsants and proton pump inhibitors) and head trauma.
- Vertigo in an older age group raises the possibility of BPPV and ischaemia of the posterior cerebral (brain-stem) circulation or the labyrinthine circulation as well as acute labyrinthitis, trauma and medication.
- Presyncope tends to be more common in older patients because of their higher prevalence of co-morbid states including heart disease, hypertension and diabetes. Medication for these conditions commonly compounds the problem as well.

Hearing loss and tinnitus

- If deafness and/or tinnitus accompanies vertigo this is strongly suggestive of pathology in the inner ear. Ménière's disease is the most common example and is particularly likely if there are recurrent episodes.
- In severe cases of acute labyrinthitis, transient hearing loss and tinnitus can also feature.
- A tumour in the cerebello-pontine angle (classically an acoustic neuroma) tends to cause progressive hearing loss and mild ataxia rather than vertigo.

Associated general medical and neurological history

Ask in particular about ischaemic heart disease and risk factors for vascular disease.

- A positive history raises the possibility of a cardiac arrhythmia or an alternative vascular event as the precipitant for vertigo or presyncope.
- Systemic infection is a common cause of presyncope especially if associated with dehydration, hypotension or pyrexia.

- Careful enquiry for additional symptoms implying brain-stem pathology is mandatory. These include diplopia, dysarthria, dysphagia, facial numbness and weakness (the facial nerve travels in close proximity to the 8th nerve in the internal auditory canal, cerebello-pontine angle and brain-stem), numbness or incoordination of a limb or limbs.
- Demyelination will be a candidate cause if there is a history of previous focal neurological symptoms.
- Ataxia is common with vertigo of both central and peripheral origin. It is also a feature of cerebellar disease and abnormalities of proprioception secondary to either peripheral nerve or dorsal column pathology. Ataxia is uncommon in presyncope.
- Presyncope is often accompanied by blurred vision, palpitation, sweating and pallor.

Anxiety and hyperventilation

Ask about the possibility of anxiety and hyperventilation. Typical symptoms include sharp chest pain, breathlessness, light-headedness and paraesthesiae around the mouth or in the tips of the fingers. Often there is a history of depression or previous panic attacks.

Family history

Enquire about a family history of vascular disease or risk factors associated with it. There may be a positive family history in Ménière's disease.

Medication history

Many medications can result in unsteadiness. Examples are anticonvulsants, antihypertensives and antidepressants. Aminoglycoside antibiotics are toxic to the vestibular nerve and can cause permanent unsteadiness. Drugs can also cause ataxia – anticonvulsants (particularly phenytoin at toxic levels) are a common example.

Substance abuse

Acute alcohol intoxication causes unsteadiness and vertigo. Sedatives, opiates, amphetamines and LSD can all cause dizziness. Chronic alcohol abuse can result in cerebellar degeneration: this is the most common cause of ataxia in the UK.

HAZARD

Acute vertigo should always raise the possibility of brain-stem or cerebellar pathology. Symptoms and signs of associated brain-stem disease must be looked for carefully because the only abnormal sign found in vestibular causes of vertigo is nystagmus, which may or may not be positional in nature. The presence of any additional focal neurological signs indicates the possibility of brain-stem or cerebellar pathology.

● Examination

Focused general and neurological examination is essential.

General examination

Look in particular for signs of cardiac disease. Check the pulse for arrhythmias such as atrial fibrillation. Listen for cardiac murmurs and check lying and standing blood pressures. A heart murmur, indicating valvular heart disease, may point to left ventricular outflow tract obstruction or perhaps mitral valve disease, both of which can be associated with vascular pathology (hypotensive or embolic) to the vestibular system or brain-stem.

Bruits in major arteries or other evidence of vascular pathology may be of relevance also in suggesting cerebrovascular disease as the cause of symptoms. Look also for signs of anaemia: skin pallor and pale conjunctivae.

Neurological examination

This is usefully systematized as follows.

Balance

- First assess for the presence of ataxia. Remember that ataxia is not found in presyncope. Truncal ataxia can be elicited by sitting the patient on the edge of the bed with feet off the ground and arms crossed in front to remove support. Unsteadiness may be spontaneous or may need to be provoked by gently pulling the patient towards you. If this is grossly normal, ask the patient to stand and examine similarly for spontaneous and provoked ataxia.
- The ataxic gait is broad-based and stumbling and will be exaggerated by asking the patient to walk with one foot in front of the other ('tandem walking'). Young, healthy adults should be able to do this both forwards and backwards without staggering.
- As previously mentioned, normal balance relies on intact visual, proprioceptive and vestibular sensory systems together with the central coordinating function of the cerebellum. It follows that cerebellar disease may result in ataxia, as will abnormalities in either vestibular or proprioceptive sensation. The latter two are especially pronounced if the pathology affecting their function is acute.
- Vision compensates for both vestibular and proprioceptive deficits, especially when the dysfunction is chronic – and this explains the importance of *Romberg's test*. This is positive if the patient becomes unsteady with eyes closed, therefore removing visual compensation for the imbalance caused by abnormal vestibular and/or proprioceptive function.

Hearing

An audiogram may be necessary but simple tests of hearing are useful also.

- Whisper numbers in the patient's ear and ask for them to be repeated.
- Rub thumb and forefinger together: a young adult should perceive this sound at arm's length. The sensitivity becomes progressively less with age, but elderly patients should still be able to sense at a distance of up to 10 cm (3 or 4 inches) from the ear.
- *Rinne's test* involves comparing the intensity of the note from a high-frequency tuning fork when it is held first in the air close to the patient's ear and then placed on the mastoid process. In conductive nerve deafness, bone conduction is better than air conduction.
- In the complementary *Weber's test*, the tuning fork is placed on the skull vertex and, normally, the sound is heard equally well in both ears. In conductive deafness the sound is heard louder in the affected ear, while in sensorineural deafness the sound is less well heard on the abnormal side.
- Deafness in association with vertigo is usually sensorineural in origin.

Fundoscopy

Examine for papilloedema, indicative of raised intracranial pressure or perhaps acute optic neuritis, retinopathy (due to diabetes or hypertension) and optic atrophy, which may indicate a previous episode of demyelination.

Cranial nerves

- **2nd, 3rd, 4th and 6th**. Gaze palsies, internuclear ophthalmoplegia (most commonly seen in demyelination) and 3rd, 4th or 6th nerve palsies will all suggest structural brain-stem disease and therefore point to a central cause for vertigo.
- **5th**. Facial numbness and/or absent corneal reflex is evidence of 5th nerve pathology and suggests a lesion in the cerebello-pontine angle.

- **7th**. Facial nerve palsy points to a structural problem in the internal auditory canal, cerebello-pontine angle or brain-stem.

Cerebellum

Cerebellar disease *per se* causes ataxia rather than vertigo, but the close anatomical association of the cerebellar and vestibular systems makes assessment crucial. Test for ataxia, dysdiadochokinesis and cerebellar speech.

Nystagmus

Nystagmus can be 'pendular' (with oscillating movements to and fro of similar amplitude, typically seen in congenital nystagmus) or 'jerk' where a slow (pathological) drift to one side is followed by a fast corrective movement.

The assessment of nystagmus is potentially complicated but a few simple rules can be applied. First differentiate between spontaneous nystagmus and provoked nystagmus, the latter being exemplified by the *Dix–Hallpike positional test* for positional nystagmus.

THINK

What is the Dix–Hallpike test?
This is a test for *benign paroxysmal positional vertigo* (BPPV). Position the patient so that when lying flat the head extends beyond the end of the examination couch. Then sit the patient upright and turn the head to 45 degrees to the right or left. Rapidly lay the patient down with the head extended. Look for nystagmus, which can take a few seconds to appear, and be aware that severe symptoms of vertigo accompany a positive test. It is virtually diagnostic of benign positional vertigo. Note that the patient will probably find this intensely unpleasant.

● Spontaneous nystagmus

- Nystagmus seen in the primary position (eyes gazing forward) is usually either congenital or secondary to acute vestibular dysfunction. The latter will be accompanied by severe systemic symptoms of nausea and vomiting in most cases.
- Nystagmus that is only apparent on eccentric gaze (ask the patient to follow a finger to one side or the other) is commonly due to cerebellar disease or perhaps drugs.
- Drug-induced nystagmus is often provoked by gaze in several different directions, although it may be maximal in one.
- Unidirectional, horizontal nystagmus does not differentiate between labyrinthine and cerebellar disease.
- Ataxic nystagmus is greater in the abducting eye and is associated with failure of adduction in the other eye. It indicates disease in the medial longitudinal fasciculus and is virtually pathognomonic of multiple sclerosis.
- Vertical nystagmus (seen on upward conjugate gaze) is diagnostic of upper brain-stem pathology (e.g. pontine infarction).
- The rare 'down-beat' nystagmus points to disease in the cervico-medullary junction and is typically seen in Arnold–Chiari malformation.

Sensory and motor systems

Test sensation and look particularly for peripheral neuropathy or loss of proprioception. Nerve fibres in the dorsal columns of the spinal cord carry the sensory modalities of proprioception (joint and position sense) and disease in this site (e.g. subacute combined degeneration of the cord) will cause disequilibrium. This is often first noticed in the dark because of visual compensation in the early stages.

Abnormal power and/or tone indicative of pyramidal tract pathology may arise with pathology in the brain-stem, but may also provide evidence of multiple site pathology in demyelination.

● Investigations

Many causes of vertigo have no confirmatory tests and the diagnosis is made on clinical grounds alone. Examples include acute labyrinthitis, Ménière's disease, vertebrobasilar migraine and hyperventilation syndrome. A CT of the head may not be sensitive enough to evaluate the course of the vestibular nerve, so MRI is the imaging modality of choice in this context.

Investigations can be approached systematically by considering the three broad classifications of dizziness. These are the basic investigations to be considered at an early stage. Other, more involved tests of autonomic function, vestibular function and audiometry will need to be considered depending on the individual circumstances and following specialist consultation.

Acute vertigo

Most blood tests in this context are done to rule out causes of presyncope or to look for evidence of infection: full blood count (FBC), erythrocyte sedimentation rate (ESR), C-reactive protein (CRP), and blood glucose. Magnetic resonance imaging (MRI) of the brain may be indicated if a clear diagnosis cannot be made on clinical grounds.

- **Positional vertigo**. Obtain an MRI of the brain to look for a posterior fossa lesion, and a Dix–Hallpike test to look for BPPV.
- **Vertigo with headache**. Obtain a CT of the head proceeding possibly to MRI of the brain to look for an intracranial space-occupying lesion.
- **Vertigo with deafness, with or without tinnitus**. Do an audiogram to define any hearing loss. Perform an MRI of the brain.

Presyncope

These tests are usual:

- FBC to look for anaemia or a raised white cell count, CRP as a marker of infection, and glucose to look for diabetes or hypoglycaemia

- ECG and ECHO to look for evidence of ischaemic or valvular cardiac disease
- 24-hour Holter monitoring to investigate for arrhythmias.

Disequilibrium

Tests may be indicated to look for a cause of any peripheral neuropathy if a cause (e.g. diabetes) is not immediately apparent. These will include tests of thyroid function and vitamin B_{12} levels, which are also required if there is any suspicion of subacute combined degeneration of the cord.

9 Acute confusion

Introduction

Acute confusion is a common medical emergency, particularly in elderly patients. It can also be referred to as 'delirium' (see **Think** below). Even in the presence of pre-existing cognitive impairment, there is usually an organic cause for an acute confusional state and a systematic search for a cause should always be undertaken. In elderly patients, acute confusion may be the only presenting symptom of disease in another organ system, such as myocardial infarction, cardiac arrhythmia, pneumonia or urosepsis.

A second important point is that acute confusion may be the first manifestation of a pathological process that can lead to a reduced level of consciousness if untreated. Examples include encephalitis and intracranial haemorrhage. Any patient presenting with confusion and a reduced level of consciousness requires urgent clinical assessment.

There are many potential causes of acute confusion. We present here a classification that aims to clarify diagnostic thinking and uses broad groupings where appropriate. We have categorized aetiology according to the age of the patient because there is a correlation of cause with age.

● Classification of confusion

Common causes of acute confusion in elderly patients

- Sepsis or acute inflammatory response, from *any* source, including:
  - Urinary tract infection
  - Pneumonia
  - Diverticulitis
  - Cholecystitis
  - Pancreatitis
- Urinary retention
- Severe constipation (also a common cause of urinary retention)
- Metabolic problems, including:
  - Electrolyte disturbance: particularly hyponatraemia, hypernatraemia, hypercalcaemia
  - Hypoglycaemia, hyperglycaemia
  - Liver failure
  - Uraemia
- Hypoxaemia, from any cause – common causes include pneumonia, exacerbation of COPD, left ventricular failure and pulmonary embolism
- Drug/toxin-induced:
  - Prescription drugs. The mechanism may be direct or indirect. Some drugs such as opiates cause confusion directly, diuretics may be responsible by causing electrolyte abnormalities. Elderly patients are more vulnerable to drug side-effects than younger patients.
  - Alcohol can cause confusion either following acute ingestion or as a result of sudden withdrawal. Confusion may herald the onset of delirium tremens
- Cardiac disease – myocardial infarction or arrhythmia of any kind

- Acute intracranial pathology, including:
  - Intracranial bleed (subdural or primary intracerebral haemorrhage)
  - Stroke
- Post-ictal state following a seizure

Common causes of acute confusion in younger patients

- Alcohol, either acute excess or withdrawal (including delirium tremens) in an alcohol-dependent patient
- Recreational drug use, particularly amphetamines, cocaine and LSD
- Severe sepsis, for example severe pneumonia
- Acute liver failure: hepatic encephalopathy
- Post-ictal state following a seizure
- Prescription drug-induced – opiates, anaesthetic agents and sedatives

Less common causes of acute confusion in any patient

- Intracranial infection – meningitis, encephalitis
- Intracranial space-occupying lesion – tumour, abscess
- Head injury, including sequelae such as an extradural haemorrhage
- Subarachnoid haemorrhage
- Cerebral (falciparum) malaria in travellers from endemic areas
- Cerebral vasculitis due, for example, to systemic lupus erythematosis (SLE)
- Hypertensive encephalopathy (rare)
- Severe hypothyroidism ('myxoedema madness') (very rare)
- Nutritional deficiency (rare in Western industrialized countries but chronic deficiency of vitamin B_{12}, thiamine and niacin can all lead to acute confusion)

💡 THINK

What are the classical features of delirium?
Delirium is an acute disturbance of consciousness, orientation, mood, cognition, speech and thought processes. It is common in hospital inpatients and mainly affects the elderly and those with a pre-existing cerebral deficit. Delirium often fluctuates in severity and is usually worst at night.

⚡ HAZARD

Delirium tremens is the most severe manifestation of acute alcohol withdrawal. It is a medical emergency and can be life-threatening. Typically, the onset occurs 2–3 days after ceasing alcohol. Features include marked visual hallucinations (often involving small creatures swarming over the bed), tremor, fever, sweating, nausea/vomiting, tachycardia, agitation and seizures.

● History

It will not be possible to obtain a meaningful history from an acutely confused patient, so you will need to gather information from other sources. A relative or friend accompanying the patient may be able to provide useful information, and telephoning the patient's general practitioner or next of kin should provide details about past medical history and prescribed medication. In addition, search the hospital's computer system for previous test results and discharge summaries. Any potential factual source should be explored and, in particular, seek details on the following.

- **Usual cognitive state**. Is the patient normally independent and lucid, or is there chronic cognitive impairment? This will provide some guidance as to the realistic goals of your management plan.

- **Medical history**. Is there a known history of any chronic condition (e.g. diabetes, cirrhosis or epilepsy)?
- **Trauma**. Has there been a recent head injury or fall? Even minor trauma in a frail elderly patient may be enough to cause a subdural haemorrhage.
- **Prescribed medications**. This is particularly important in elderly patients. If the information is not immediately available from an accompanying relative or friend, other sources should be explored, including those suggested above. In particular, enquire about sedatives, opioid analgesics, neuroleptics and anticonvulsant drugs.
- **Alcohol intake**. Ask about usual and recent intake. Elderly patients often conceal the extent of their alcohol intake from relatives (and doctors!) and you may need to keep an open mind about the truthfulness of the reported alcohol intake.
- **Recreational drug use**. Is there a history of recent or past drug abuse? Many patients (and their accompanying friends) may not admit to this initially.
- **History of recent illness**. Is there any suggestion of symptoms of infection (e.g. cough, fever or dysuria), abdominal pain or headache before the onset of confusion?
- **Recent travel history**. Has the patient returned from overseas recently, particularly from a malaria endemic area?

● Examination

If no accompanying friend, relative or carer is available you may be examining a confused patient before having been able to obtain a history. Clinical examination can be challenging in itself, because confused patients are often non-compliant; but much information can still be obtained as discussed in Chapter 7 on seizures. Bearing in mind the causes of acute confusion, look in particular for signs of the following.

- **Sepsis**. Is the patient febrile, hypotensive, tachypnoeic, tachycardic or coughing, or is there an aroma of foul-smelling urine? Auscultate the chest for crackles, bronchial breathing or wheezing suggestive of respiratory or cardiac pathology. Examine the abdomen for signs of peritonitis: guarding, rigidity or absent bowel sounds.
- **Hypoxia**. Examine for tachypnoea or central cyanosis.
- **Head injury**. Look for scalp lacerations and facial bruising.
- **Alcohol excess**. Does the patient smell of alcohol, indicating acute intoxication, or is a hepatic foetor present, indicating possible hepatic encephalopathy?
- **Urinary retention**. Look for suprapubic tenderness and a palpable distended bladder.
- **Drug abuse**. Examine for needle track marks.
- **Meningism**. Examine for photophobia and a stiff neck. A genuinely photophobic patient will cover the eyes completely in a well-lit emergency department. To look for evidence of neck stiffness, ask the patient whether he or she can 'put their chin on their chest'. If they can, then they do not have neck stiffness. If the patient is too confused to be able to cooperate with this, attempt to flex the neck gently with the patient supine. A stiff neck will be immediately evident if present. If you think the patient may have meningitis (in other words, there are signs of meningism and sepsis), then look carefully for the typical non-blanching purpuric rash of *Meningococcus*. If you find it, call for senior help immediately.

HAZARD

If you find signs of meningism, administer broad-spectrum antibiotics immediately to cover the possibility of bacterial meningitis before proceeding with the rest of the clinical assessment.

- **Chronic liver disease**. Examine for spider naevi, palmar erythema, leuconychia, ascites, bruising and bleeding into the skin, poor nutrition and muscle wasting. The presence of such signs raises the possibility of hepatic encephalopathy or delirium tremens as the cause of confusion.

- **Post-ictal state**. A clue to this includes the presence of lateral tongue lacerations from tongue biting during a seizure.

- **Neurological deficit**. Perform as complete a neurological examination as you can. Document the level of consciousness (e.g. using the Glasgow Coma Scale), the presence of spontaneous limb movement, pupillary reflexes, limb tone and reflexes. In addition examine the fundi to look for papilloedema and other abnormalities. Good patient cooperation is required to accurately document power, sensation, coordination and cranial nerve examination. Obvious asymmetry in pupil size, limb tone, reflexes or movement may point towards significant intracranial pathology such as a stroke, space-occupying lesion or intracranial bleed.

- **Malignant hypertension**. If there is marked hypertension (e.g. diastolic >140 mmHg), this may indicate malignant hypertension. Other features of malignant hypertension include renal failure and papilloedema.

- **Mini-mental test score**. A brief measure of the degree of confusion on presentation can be very helpful, particularly if it can be repeated to assess clinical progress. An example of such an assessment tool is the Mini-Mental Test which is scored out of 10.

THINK

What are the components of the 10-point Mini-Mental Test?

- Age – must be correct.
- Time, without looking at a clock or watch – must be correct to the nearest hour.

- Address to remember (e.g. 42 West Street) – given as a test of immediate memory and retested at the end.
- Month – must be exact.
- Year – must be exact, except in January or February when last year is OK.
- Name of place or type of place or town – 'in hospital' is insufficient.
- Date of birth – must be exact.
- Start of WW1or WW2 – must be exact, 1914 or 1939.
- Name of present monarch or prime minister.
- Counting backwards from 20 to 0 – must be completely correct.

Then re-check the 'address to remember'.

● Investigations

Bedside tests

A number of simple investigations that can be performed at the bedside will aid diagnosis of acute confusion.

- *Blood glucose.* This can be measured from fingerprick testing. Hypoglycaemia must be treated immediately with intravenous dextrose.
- *Pulse oximetry.* If the patient is hypoxic, administer oxygen immediately and perform arterial blood gas analysis looking for acid–base disturbance and evidence of respiratory failure. Underlying possible diagnoses such as pneumonia, exacerbation of chronic obstructive pulmonary disease (COPD), left ventricular failure and pulmonary embolism should be investigated further in hypoxic patients.
- *Blood biochemistry*:
  - serum urea and electrolytes, looking in particular at the sodium and urea levels in the confused patient
  - serum C-reactive protein (CRP), looking for evidence of an acute inflammatory response or sepsis

- serum calcium
- random blood glucose, which should be requested in addition to fingerprick testing
- liver function tests, looking for evidence of chronic liver disease.

- *Full blood count.* If the patient is febrile, check the white cell and neutrophil counts.
- *Blood cultures.* Send these with any confused febrile patient.
- *Urine dipstick and MSU for culture.* The presence of protein, leucocytes, blood and nitrites indicates possible urinary tract infection, a very common cause of confusion in the elderly patient.
- *ECG.* Look for evidence of arrhythmia or acute coronary syndrome. Arrhythmias such as rapid atrial fibrillation and complete heart block are well-documented causes of acute confusion in elderly patients.
- *Malarial parasites.* In a febrile, confused patient with a recent history of travel to a malaria endemic area, send several blood samples for a thick film to look for malarial parasites. A single negative result does not exclude the diagnosis.

Radiological investigations

- *Chest x-ray.* Perform this in all confused patients, looking mainly for evidence of infection or cardiac failure. Beware of the limitations of a poor-quality portable CXR in an uncooperative patient who cannot remain still (see **Hazard** below).
- *CT of head.* This is indicated if no obvious cause for confusion has been identified from the bedside and laboratory investigations listed above. It is a mandatory investigation if there is reduced consciousness. A CT without intravenous contrast enhancement will pick up most cases of intracranial bleeding, and CT with contrast will pick up space-occupying lesions. See Chapter 10 for a fuller discussion of the technical aspects.

HAZARD

Patients who are unable to cooperate adequately with the radiographer in obtaining a good-quality postero-anterior (PA) CXR will usually have a sitting or supine antero-posterior (AP) film performed. AP films obtained in sick patients are often of poor quality and it is important to understand the limitations this imposes on interpretation. Inexperienced staff often over-interpret apparent abnormalities that are, in fact, artefacts arising from the poor technical quality of the film. Common examples include the cardiac shadow and mediastinum looking abnormally wide on an AP film, and the hila looking more prominent if the film is rotated. Obtain a report from an expert and, if there is any doubt about the appearance, request a repeat PA CXR as soon as the patient is sufficiently recovered.

Additional investigations

Infection

If initial examination and investigations suggest an acute inflammatory response or sepsis, identifying the source of infection is the next important step. As already stated, the most common sources of sepsis causing acute infection are the urinary tract and lungs. If initial investigations do not support either of these as the source (negative urine dipstick and normal chest x-ray), look elsewhere for infection.

- **Intra-abdominal sepsis or inflammation**. Possibilities include cholecystitis, diverticulitis, pancreatitis, ischaemic bowel or a liver abscess.
- **Intracranial infection** (meningitis, encephalitis) – or other intracranial pathology.

Further investigations may then be required, as follows.

- *Abdominal ultrasound*. This can assess liver architecture reliably and diagnose bile duct dilation. It does have limitations, however, and is not good at assessing the pancreas for example.
- *CT of abdomen and pelvis*. This provides more accurate imaging of intra-abdominal organs than ultrasound. Intravenous contrast is required, which carries the potential for causing renal impairment in sick patients who are poorly hydrated or who have pre-existing renal disease. In addition, an acutely confused patient may require sedation to ensure images of satisfactory quality.
- *Serum amylase or lipase* (depending on which is performed in your local laboratory). Elevated levels are found in pancreatitis – usually at least five times the upper level of normal. Note, however, that most causes of an 'acute abdomen' can result in a raised amylase or lipase, particularly a perforated upper abdominal viscus.
- *CT of the head* (as described above).
- *Lumbar puncture* – to obtain cerebrospinal fluid (CSF) for analysis. This should be performed if meningitis or encephalitis is suspected. In acute confusion, an urgent CT of the head should be performed before embarking on a lumbar puncture, to assess the possibility of raised intracranial pressure. A full description of CSF analysis and the findings associated with intracranial infection can be found in Chapter 10.

Hypoxia

If the patient is hypoxic, consider the differential diagnoses of pneumonia, left ventricular failure (LVF), exacerbation of COPD and pulmonary embolism (PE).

- A good quality CXR should detect or exclude pneumonia and LVF.
- Exacerbation of COPD is generally evident on clinical examination (e.g. pronounced wheezing).

- If no immediate cause for hypoxia is apparent on initial investigations, the CXR does not show a significant abnormality and the patient is not septic, consider the possibility of a PE. This topic is covered in more detail in the chapters on chest pain and breathlessness, but the investigation of choice is then a CT pulmonary angiogram.

CLINICAL TIP

Systematic investigation of an acute confusional state should lead to a cause being identified within a few hours in most cases. In frail, elderly patients, it is common to find more than one contributory factor, each of which will require consideration in your management plan.

10 Acute headache

● Introduction

Most adults experience an acute headache at some point during their life. The majority of acute headaches are benign and self-limiting, but a minority herald the onset of a life-threatening neurological condition. Headache is also a common symptom of many non-neurological conditions (e.g. influenza). The diagnostic skill resides in distinguishing the minority with significant pathology from the majority with self-limiting headache. Adopting a systematic approach with attention first to symptoms and signs of serious conditions will help in quickly ruling in (or out) significant pathology.

● History

Some simple initial questions will indicate immediately that you are dealing with a life-threatening situation.

Has there been an episode of loss of consciousness?
Sudden loss of consciousness occurs in half of all patients sustaining a subarachnoid haemorrhage (SAH) and it often lasts for more than one hour.

● Classification of acute headache

Vascular

- Subarachnoid haemorrhage (SAH). In patients presenting to emergency departments with acute severe headache, this is the main differential diagnosis requiring investigation.
- Intracerebral haemorrhage.
- Subdural haemorrhage (SDH). Risk factors for an SDH include old age, alcohol excess and anticoagulation therapy. There is often a history of a recent fall or head injury but the trauma may have been so insignificant as not to be remembered.
- Extradural haemorrhage. This is caused by a head injury resulting in a skull fracture which tears the middle meningeal artery. It is immediately life-threatening.
- Temporal arteritis. This typically causes headache with unilateral tenderness over the temporal artery. It is rare in patients aged under 50 years.

Migraine

This is a common cause of severe headache presenting to emergency services.

Muscular

Tension headache ('stress'). This is very common. Tight, sore neck muscles are often evident and a recurrent history is common.

Meningeal irritation

- Bacterial meningitis. Causative organisms include *Neisseria meningitidis*, *Streptococcus* species and *Mycobacterium tuberculosis*. This is an extreme medical emergency.
- Viral meningitis. Causes include herpes simplex (HSV), enteroviruses (such as Coxsackie virus and Echovirus), HIV, Epstein–Barr virus (EBV) and cytomegalovirus (CMV).

- Viral 'meningism'. A headache with some photophobia can be one manifestation of a viral illness in patients with 'flu-like' symptoms.
- Encephalitis. There is often some adjacent meningeal inflammation in patients with encephalitis. The most common causes are viruses. Examples in developed countries include HSV, enteroviruses, mumps, EBV, herpes zoster, adenovirus and influenza. There are also many rarer endemic causes of encephalitis in specific regions of the world.

Raised intracranial pressure

- Primary intracerebral tumours. Examples include gliomas and astrocytomas.
- Brain metastases. Tumours that commonly metastasize to the brain include breast, lung and melanoma. Brain metastases are much more common than primary intracerebral tumours.
- Cerebral abscess. These are now rare in developed countries. Don't forget that cerebral tuberculomas are still common in developing countries with a high incidence of tuberculosis (TB).
- Colloid cyst. This rare tumour can cause recurrent severe headaches if situated in the third ventricle, obstructing the flow of cerebrospinal fluid (CSF).
- Malignant hypertension. This is an uncommon clinical syndrome caused by severe progressive hypertension with a diastolic blood pressure >140 mmHg. The syndrome includes renal failure and papilloedema and may be associated with encephalopathy and seizures. Note that uncomplicated hypertension does not cause headaches.
- Benign intracranial hypertension. This condition is mainly seen in young obese women. Classically, papilloedema is present in association with visual disturbance.

- Intracranial venous thrombosis. This is rare and can be associated with thrombophilia, severe intercurrent illness and sinus or intracranial infection. The exact presentation depends on which venous sinus is thrombosed. (A detailed discussion of this is beyond the scope of this text.)

Drug- or toxin-induced

- GTN/nitrates. Headache is a common side-effect of nitrates.
- Carbon monoxide poisoning. This cause of headaches is often overlooked.

Carbon dioxide retention due to respiratory failure

This commonly causes early morning headaches as a result of overnight hypercapnia leading to cerebral vasodilatation. Respiratory conditions which cause this include:

- Obstructive sleep apnoea
- Obesity hypoventilation syndrome
- Respiratory failure due to neuromuscular or chest wall disease such as motor neurone disease or severe scoliosis.

Infections in general

- Pneumonia
- Influenza
- Common cold
- Malaria

Miscellaneous

- Post-coital headache
- Acute glaucoma
- Sinusitis
- Cluster headache. This is an uncommon and specific syndrome mainly affecting young men. The classical history is of being woken at night with a severe

unilateral headache and eye pain which lasts for several hours. Nasal congestion, lacrimation and vomiting are also common
- Herpes zoster ('shingles') of cervical nerve roots
- Post lumbar puncture
- Carotid artery dissection. This is an unusual cause of stroke and can cause unilateral neck/head pain
- Altitude sickness (this only applies if the subject is at an altitude of over about 3000 m).

Are there symptoms of meningism?

Ask about photophobia and neck stiffness. Symptoms of meningism increase the likelihood of diagnoses such as meningitis (bacterial or viral), subarachnoid haemorrhage and encephalitis. Note that the history in most of these cases will be short (hours rather than days) and, in the case of SAH, meningism usually takes more than three hours to develop. A longer history (days to weeks) with symptoms of meningitis should prompt consideration of meningeal tuberculosis (TB), particularly in patients born in countries with a high incidence of TB.

⚡ HAZARD

Bacterial meningitis is one of the most extreme medical emergencies that the majority of doctors will ever see. The classical description of a stiff neck can be an understatement – patients with established bacterial meningitis may lie rigidly still and resist all movement. Give intravenous antibiotics **immediately** if you suspect bacterial meningitis. Never delay treatment to wait for the results of investigations as this may make the difference between life and death.

Has there been a head injury in the past few days or weeks?
This increases the risk of subdural haemorrhage (SDH) or extradural haemorrhage. In an elderly person, a simple fall may be sufficient to cause such complications. Remember also that a head injury may not be remembered if the patient was intoxicated at the time.

HAZARD

Always consider the possibility of an extradural haemorrhage in a patient with a headache who reports a head injury at any time in the preceding hours or days. Typically the subject recovers quickly after the initial injury and then develops headache and reduced consciousness perhaps with hemiparesis hours to days later. Urgent neurosurgery is required to save the life of any patient with an extradural haemorrhage.

Does the patient have a reduced conscious level?
This is a 'red flag' sign in a patient presenting with a headache. It indicates a higher likelihood of life-threatening conditions such as meningitis, encephalitis, intracranial bleeding of any kind, raised intracranial pressure and carbon monoxide poisoning.

THINK

What 'red flag' symptoms and signs should one be aware of in any patient presenting with acute headache? Altered consciousness, symptoms of raised intracranial pressure, signs of sepsis, recent head injury and sudden onset of 'worst headache ever'.

Are there recent symptoms of raised intracranial pressure?

These include headaches that are worst on waking and exacerbated by bending forward, coughing or straining at stool. Ask this particularly of patients presenting with headache who have a past history of a malignancy which is known to metastasize to the brain.

Is this the worst headache the patient has ever experienced?

A 'worst ever' headache in a patient not normally prone to headaches should prompt further investigation for conditions such as subarachnoid haemorrhage.

HAZARD

Over-reliance on the classical textbook descriptions of the presenting features of SAH can lead to the diagnosis being missed in some cases. This is important as SAH carries a mortality of 50 per cent, and 30 per cent of survivors do not regain their independence. Note that only about half of patients with SAH describe the classical explosive sudden-onset headache. In the other half the headache can evolve over several minutes. Other diagnostic clues to SAH include sudden loss of consciousness, which occurs in 50 per cent of patients. Vomiting occurs in 70 per cent but is not specific to SAH – it is common in migraine, for example. Conversely a headache lasting under an hour makes SAH unlikely.

What was the mode of onset?

A headache with a very sudden onset is suspicious of a vascular event such as SAH or intracerebral bleeding. The headache of SAH is often described in texts as a 'blow to the back of the head' but the salient feature of the headache in many cases is that it is sudden and catastrophic – the worst headache the patient has ever had. Note, however, that a significant minority of patients with SAH do not describe sudden onset of headache – it may evolve over several minutes.

Does the patient suffer regularly with headaches?

Tension headaches and migraine tend to be recurrent events. If the patient is prone to such headaches, ask whether this one is different in any way. Some patterns of migraine have very typical features and there is often a preceding visual aura followed by a unilateral headache. Nausea and vomiting are common.

Regular morning headaches in obese patients should prompt consideration of obstructive sleep apnoea or overnight hypoventilation. Frequent headaches in obese young women can be due to benign intracranial hypertension. Regular headaches and grogginess can also be a symptom of carbon monoxide poisoning: ask whether other household members are affected and whether there is a gas heater or boiler operating in the patient's home.

Is the headache unilateral?

A number of causes of headache tend to cause unilateral symptoms. These include migraine, cluster headache, temporal arteritis, glaucoma, sinusitis and herpes zoster of the scalp ('shingles').

Is there associated visual disturbance?

- Visual disturbance with an 'aura' is a common precursor of a migrainous headache. Examples include flashing lights or 'zigzags' of light and the appearance of a temporary scotoma or hemianopia.
- Visual disturbance is a feature of glaucoma, resulting in blurred and impaired vision in the affected eye.
- In a patient with suspected temporal arteritis, visual disturbance is an emergency indicating impending loss of sight due to involvement of ocular blood vessels.
- Visual disturbance occurs in benign intracranial hypertension when it is due to severe papilloedema.

Does the patient have any intercurrent illness?
Headache is a common symptom of many upper respiratory tract viral infections as well as pneumonia.

Is there a history of recent foreign travel?
Travel to an area where malaria or endemic encephalitis is prevalent may be significant.

THINK

When should one consider the endemic forms of encephalitis seen in some parts of the world?
If you suspect encephalitis, always ask about recent travel and take advice from a consultant microbiologist as to local known causative viruses. Endemic forms include Japanese encephalitis in SE Asia, West Nile virus in East Africa (and recently recorded in New York, USA) and Ross River virus in Australia.

Drug history
Note whether the patient has recently started isosorbide mononitrate therapy.

● Examination

- Look for evidence of sepsis. Is the patient febrile, hypotensive or shocked? If so, then diagnoses such as meningitis and pneumonia are more likely.
- Look for signs of meningism such as photophobia or a stiff neck. A genuinely photophobic patient will cover their eyes completely in a well-lit emergency department or request that all lights be switched off. Ask the patient whether they can 'put their chin on their chest'. If they can, then they do not have neck stiffness. If the patient is unable to cooperate with your examination (for instance if they are semi-conscious and lying supine) then attempt to lift the head

gently off the bed. A stiff neck will be immediately evident if present. If you find signs of meningism, give intravenous broad-spectrum antibiotics immediately to cover the possibility of bacterial meningitis before proceeding with the rest of your assessment (see **Hazard** above). Note that patients with migraine often prefer a darkened room without exhibiting frank signs of meningism.

- If you think the patient may have meningitis (there are signs of meningism, sepsis or altered consciousness), look carefully for the typical non-blanching purpuric rash of *Meningococcus*. If you find it, call for senior help immediately.

- Assess the degree of consciousness. Recording the Glasgow Coma Score is helpful (see Table 2.1 in Chapter 2, p. 19). Any impairment is a 'red flag' sign as described above in the History section.

- Perform a full neurological examination, including the cranial nerves. Any new focal deficit usually indicates serious pathology, although some rarer forms of migraine can cause temporary neurological deficits, which resolve within 24 hours.

- Perform fundoscopy looking for papilloedema. If present, the patient has raised intracranial pressure requiring urgent investigation. If the patient is photophobic then fundoscopy will be impossible, and it is very challenging to perform adequate fundoscopy anyway in a busy, well-lit emergency department.

- If the headache is unilateral:
  - Examine the patient for tenderness over the frontal and maxillary sinuses as tenderness at these sites indicates likely acute sinusitis.
  - Look carefully at the scalp for lesions of herpes zoster.
  - In patients over 50, palpate the temporal arteries for tenderness. If present, this may indicate a diagnosis of temporal arteritis.
  - Look at the pupils. A red eye with unilateral headache requires an urgent ophthalmological opinion looking for acute glaucoma.

● Investigations

There is no diagnostic test for migraine or tension headache. These are essentially clinical diagnoses supported where necessary by negative investigations for more serious pathology. The presence of any of the 'red flag' features described earlier should prompt an urgent request for a CT of the head.

Radiological investigations

Many of the most life-threatening causes of acute headache can be quickly ruled in or out by means of a CT scan of the head. This can be done with or without injection of radiological contrast. Usual practice is to perform a scan without contrast, proceeding to a second scan with contrast if no intracerebral bleeding is identified on the first scan. Diagnoses that can usually be made confidently with non-contrast CT are:

● subarachnoid haemorrhage
● intracerebral haemorrhage (Fig. 10.1)
● subdural haemorrhage
● extradural haemorrhage
● colloid cyst.

CLINICAL TIP

Note that the diagnostic yield on CT is maximal at 98 per cent in the first 24 hours following a subarachnoid haemorrhage. It drops to 86 per cent at 48 hours and to 76 per cent at five days. A lumbar puncture (see below) is therefore required to exclude SAH if the patient presents more than 24 hours after the onset of symptoms.

Space-occupying lesions such as a cerebral tumour or abscess will usually manifest as an area of cerebral oedema or asymmetry on a non-contrast CT scan. Repeating the scan with contrast will usually delineate such lesions clearly with

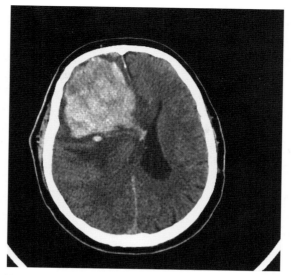

Fig. 10.1 Non-contrast computerized tomography scan showing a huge primary intracerebral haemorrhage in the right frontal region

'ring enhancement'. Diagnoses that can be confirmed with contrast-enhanced CT are:

- cerebral tumours, both primary and metastatic (Fig. 10.2)
- cerebral abscess, including tuberculomas.

There are less specific abnormalities that can be detected by CT of the head. They include the following:

- raised intracranial pressure (for instance due to benign intracranial hypertension or malignant hypertension), with reduction in the size of the ventricles and effacement of the cerebral sulci
- non-specific areas of low attenuation, which can be seen in some cases of encephalitis but are not diagnostic.

Note that it is *not* possible to diagnose any of the other causes of acute headache that are discussed in this chapter on a CT scan of the head. Any non-specific abnormalities picked up by CT will need to be further clarified with magnetic resonance

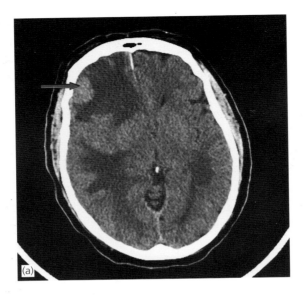

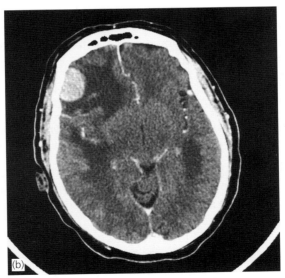

Fig. 10.2 (a) Non-contrast computerized tomography scan showing a cerebral metastasis (arrowed) with surrounding oedema. (b) The same patient after injection of radiological contrast. The metastasis is now much more clearly delineated

imaging of the brain. MRI may also show non-specific abnormalities in patients with encephalitis, and occasionally the pattern may be typical of a particular organism (e.g. temporal lobe changes in herpes simplex encephalitis). However, even the MRI may not give a precise diagnosis.

Finally, always obtain a chest x-ray in a febrile patient with an acute headache. The diagnosis may be pneumonia.

Laboratory tests

- *Full blood count.* Look for evidence of infection such as a raised neutrophil count. Remember that non-neurological infection such as pneumonia can present with acute headache.
- *Blood cultures.* Send these if there is any possibility of bacterial meningitis.
- *Blood film for malarial parasites.* Request this in any patient who has returned from a malarial area in the previous few weeks. Do not rely on one negative result to exclude malaria unless you have clearly identified an alternative cause for the patient's symptoms. It is good practice to send several blood films in cases where malaria is a possibility.
- *Viral serology.* Consider this in any patient in whom a diagnosis of viral meningitis or encephalitis is a possibility. Take advice from a microbiologist or infectious diseases specialist about the specific viruses you should test for.
- *Erythrocyte sedimentation rate* (ESR). Check this in patients aged over 50 in whom temporal arteritis is a possibility. A normal result effectively excludes the diagnosis and the ESR is usually markedly raised (over 100) in cases of temporal arteritis.
- *Carboxyhaemoglobin level* (if carbon monoxide poisoning is suspected). This test needs to be done as soon as possible because levels quickly reduce after the patient is removed from the source of CO. A normal level does not therefore exclude the diagnosis. A CO level above 10 per cent is definitely abnormal.

Examination of the cerebrospinal fluid by lumbar puncture

Lumbar puncture

A lumbar puncture (LP) is indicated if you suspect any of the following diagnoses:

- meningitis
- encephalitis
- a strong clinical suspicion of subarachnoid haemorrhage with a normal CT of the head, particularly if the patient has presented more than 24 hours after the onset of headache
- benign intracranial hypertension.

In practice a CT is often performed before an LP in order to 'rule out' evidence of raised intracranial pressure, but this is necessary only in certain circumstances (see **Think** below).

Examination of the CSF

Opening pressure

Measure this first with a manometer (supplied with most LP kits) before collecting CSF. The normal opening pressure in adults is $< 15\,mmHg$ or $< 15\,cmH_2O$.

- Patients with meningitis will have a degree of raised intracranial pressure together with other CSF abnormalities described below.
- Patients with benign intracranial hypertension have raised pressure ($> 25\,mmHg$ or $> 25\,cmH_2O$) but with otherwise normal CSF.

Clarity and appearance

Normal CSF is clear and colourless.

- In viral meningitis and encephalitis the appearance will be clear.
- In bacterial meningitis the CSF may look cloudy.

- More than 12 hours after a subarachnoid haemorrhage the CSF may exhibit a yellow tinge known as xanthochromia (caused by breakdown of bilirubin from red blood cells). Xanthochromia is often not visible to the naked eye, so examination in the laboratory using spectrophotometry is required to detect this. Xanthochromia is maximal 12 hours to 14 days after an SAH and its presence declines thereafter.
- Blood-stained CSF is usually due to a 'bloody tap' (bleeding from the LP procedure itself) but may indicate SAH. Ask your laboratory to spin it down to look for xanthochromia if clinical suspicion of SAH is high.

THINK

Is the presence of blood in the CSF always significant? Red blood cells (RBCs) are often present in small quantities in the CSF, usually due to bleeding from the lumbar puncture. Classical teaching advises that three bottles of CSF be collected and numbered sequentially. Then a declining number of RBCs in each sequential bottle is said to indicate a 'bloody tap' rather than SAH. However, this is not an entirely reliable way to rule out SAH; xanthochromia should always be looked for by spectrophotometry.

Protein level

A normal level is 0.2–0.4 g/L.

- Levels are slightly elevated in viral meningitis and encephalitis (raised but usually under 1 g/L).
- In bacterial meningitis the level is often above 1 g/L.
- In tuberculous meningitis the CSF protein is usually grossly elevated (in the experience of one of the authors, up to 11 g/L).

Cell count

Normal CSF contains no cells. The presence of polymorphs (white cells) suggests infection: in viral meningitis, encephalitis and tuberculous meningitis lymphocytes are usually predominant. In bacterial meningitis neutrophils will be dominant. Red blood cells are often present in small quantities in CSF – see **Think** above for the significance of this finding.

Glucose level

In normal CSF the glucose level is about 50–60 per cent of the blood glucose level. Viral infections usually do not affect the CSF glucose but bacterial infections cause it to drop. Bacterial meningitis causes the CSF glucose to drop below 50 per cent of the blood level, and tuberculous meningitis usually causes a very profound drop in CSF glucose.

CLINICAL TIP

Collating the results of the CSF examination will often reveal a pattern of abnormality that leads to the probable diagnosis. These patterns are summarized in Table 10.1.

Table 10.1 Cerebrospinal fluid findings helpful in differential diagnosis

	Normal	Viral meningitis or encephalitis	Bacterial meningitis	Tuberculous meningitis	SAH
Opening pressure	<15 mmHg	Raised	Raised	Raised	Raised
Appearance	Clear	Clear	Cloudy	May be cloudy	Xanthochromia
Cell count	Nil	Mainly lymphocytes	Mainly neutrophils	Mainly lymphocytes	May see red cells present
Protein level	0.2–0.4 g/L	Slightly up, often <1 g/L	Raised >1 g/L	Grossly raised, often >2 g/L	Normal
Glucose	50–60% blood value	Near normal	<50% blood value	Often very low	Normal

SAH, subarachnoid haemorrhage

THINK

Should one request a CT of the head before embarking on a lumbar puncture in every case?

This is a contentious issue. In patients with significantly raised intracranial pressure, the risk is that an LP will lead to herniation of the brain into the foramen magnum (known as 'coning'). CT is often done to look for a 'mass effect' or evidence of raised intracranial pressure in an attempt to quantify this potential risk. If you have quick access to a CT of the head then it should ideally be done first before proceeding to an LP. If you do not have quick access, then it is usually safe to proceed directly to LP providing none of the following are present: confusion, focal neurological signs, papilloedema, a recent seizure or immunosuppression.

Other tests

Early-morning blood gas measurement is helpful if there is a suspicion that hypercapnia may be the cause of morning headache in a patient with a history suspicious of sleep apnoea or respiratory failure. A referral to a respiratory or sleep specialist will also be indicated for further investigation with formal sleep studies.

11 Weakness

● Introduction

Weakness can be a manifestation of neurological disease, primary muscle disease or generalized metabolic or electrolyte abnormalities. When assessing the patient who presents with weakness, approaching the problem anatomically as well as pathologically will assist you in constructing a differential diagnosis.

The fundamental clue to the anatomical site of the lesion is the distribution of weakness. For example, hemiparesis is highly likely to be caused by a lesion either high in the pyramidal tract or in the contralateral motor cortex. The potential site of a lesion causing paraparesis is, however, more variable, ranging from the motor cortex para-sagitally (i.e. extending across the midline to affect both left and right cortices) through spinal cord pathology to problems at the nerve root or peripheral nerve level. Guillain–Barré syndrome is an example of the latter.

A further critical distinction to be made is between upper motor neurone (UMN) weakness and lower motor neurone (LMN) weakness. UMN weakness will be caused by abnormalities of the motor cortex or pyramidal tracts and LMN weakness will arise from diseases affecting the 'motor unit', which comprises the motor neurone in the anterior horn of the spinal cord, its axon, the neuromuscular junction and the muscle fibres innervated by that axon.

● Classification of weakness

Is there objective, neurological weakness?

If the answer is 'no', consider:
- Anaemia
- Chronic infection
- Malignancy
- Chronic cardiac or respiratory disease
- Depression
- Deconditioning

If the answer is 'yes', ask the following.

Is weakness generalized or localized?

If the answer is 'generalized', consider:
- Myasthenia gravis (worse with exertion)
- Cachexia
- Metabolic abnormalities (note that most of these are rare): mitochondrial diseases, glycogen disorders – McArdle's syndrome, familial periodic paralysis, severe hypokalaemia from other causes

If the answer is 'localized', move on to the following:

What is the distribution of the weakness, asymmetric or symmetric?

If the answer is 'asymmetric', consider:
- Hemiparesis or monoparesis – highly suggestive of cortical (the most common cause being embolic or thrombotic stroke), brain-stem or, rarely, spinal cord disease
- Paraparesis – spinal cord compression, anterior spinal artery occlusion, transverse myelitis, intramedullary tumour (note that the paraparesis of spinal cord disease may be symmetric or asymmetric)
- Nerve root compression
- Cauda equina compression
- Mononeuropathy or mononeuritis multiplex
- Primary muscle disease – disuse atrophy

If the answer is 'symmetrical', proceed to the following:

What is the pattern of weakness?

- Specific distribution:
  - Muscular dystrophy
  - Hereditary neuropathy: Charcot–Marie–Tooth disease
  - Myasthenia gravis
  - Inflammatory polyneuropathy: Guillain–Barré syndrome and its variants
- Proximal distribution:
  - Myopathy due, for example, to long-term corticosteroid use
  - Duchenne muscular dystrophy
  - Myasthenia gravis
- Distal distribution:
  - Peripheral neuropathy
  - Motor neurone disease
  - Myasthenia gravis
  - Myotonic dystrophy

Possible pathology

Combine this anatomical approach with enquiry as to possible pathology:

- Vascular
- Infective
- Neoplastic
- Degenerative, especially due to spinal arthritis or disc pathology
- Demyelinating
- Inflammatory from other causes, such as granulomatous disease, vasculitis or connective tissue disease

The speed of onset of weakness is the cardinal clue to pathological aetiology. A sudden onset will suggest a vascular cause leading to acute neurological damage, whereas a more gradual onset is likely in more slowly progressive pathological processes such as primary muscle disease, extrinsic cord compression or secondary to an intracerebral tumour. Weakness resulting from demyelinating diseases can present with varying degrees of suddenness.

> **HAZARD**
>
> It is vital to assess a patient's subjective complaints accurately; the medical meaning of the term 'weakness' is a reduction in strength, but patients may not use it in this way. Fatigue is often confused with weakness and many non-neurological problems may present with this complaint. It is important to consider and exclude them. Some examples are: fatigue; sleep disorders; clinical depression; anaemia; chronic heart failure; chronic renal failure; abnormal sensation or coordination (both of which may be confused with weakness) and stiffness (e.g. the rigidity associated with Parkinson's disease).

● History

A systematic approach employing the following steps should prove useful.

Non-neurological diagnoses masquerading as weakness

Consider non-neurological diagnoses as mentioned in the **Hazard** box above.

Distribution of weakness

Direct questioning of particular functional movements will assist in localizing a particular distribution of genuine neurological weakness – but this does not preclude the importance of allowing the patient to elaborate on his or her functional deficit.

- Difficulty with zips and buttons or with door handles points to a problem with a distal upper limb. So does a complaint of deteriorating handwriting.
- Problems with putting on a shirt or a jacket and difficulty with combing hair suggest proximal weakness in an upper limb.
- Distal lower limb weakness classically produces complaints of tripping while walking (weak ankle dorsiflexors), difficulty with running (weak ankle plantar flexors) and unsteadiness when walking over rough ground.
- Typical complaints of proximal lower limb weakness include difficulty in rising from a chair (particularly a low chair) or in climbing out of the bath. Gluteal muscle weakness is especially noticed by patients on climbing stairs and quadriceps weakness on descending stairs.

Upper motor neurone or lower motor neurone?

The critical distinction between upper and lower motor neurone pathology will rely to a large extent on the examination findings, but the distribution of weakness from the clinical history is also informative.

Monoparesis

Global weakness of a single limb (monoparesis) is difficult to explain on the basis of LMN pathology apart from trauma, and it is virtually diagnostic of upper motor neurone disease. Neuro-anatomical considerations explain that contralateral monoparesis can result from a localized lesion in the motor cortex (Fig. 11.1a) and from an ipsilateral lesion in the spinal cord below the neck. In the latter instance, however, there is likely to be dissociated sensory loss as well (ipsilateral dorsal column loss of proprioception and contralateral spinothalamic loss of pain and temperature (Fig. 11.1b).

Hemiparesis

Contralateral hemiparesis is likely to be caused by a lesion deep in the cerebral hemisphere near the internal capsule, where the

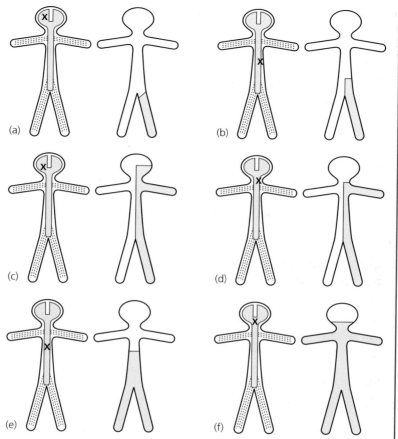

Fig. 11.1 Anatomical sites of lesions responsible for various patterns of weakness (see text). Reproduced with permission from Wilkinson I and Lennox G, *Essential Neurology*, 4th edn (Wiley Blackwell, 2005)

concentration of fibre pathways is likely to cause disruption of motor fibres to the whole of one side of the body, including the face, as well as causing contralateral sensory abnormalities and visual disturbance (homonymous hemianopia) (Fig. 11.1c).

Ipsilateral hemiparesis may result from a unilateral high cervical cord lesion. The face will be spared and there is likely to be dissociated sensory loss as described above (Fig 11.1d).

Paraparesis

This can be explained anatomically by either upper (below the cervical part of the cord, Fig. 11.1e) or lower motor neurone pathology, but this devastating medical emergency must be considered to be due to cord compression until proved otherwise (see **Hazard** below).

Quadriparesis

This results from a spinal cord lesion in the upper cervical cord or brain-stem (Fig. 11.1f).

⚡ HAZARD

Speedy diagnosis of spinal cord compression together with urgent management to relieve it is one of the crucial lessons of acute medicine. Functional recovery from cord compression is directly related to the speed with which it is relieved, and residual paraparesis or paraplegia is a devastating potential outcome for the patient.

- Consider that paraparesis is due to spinal cord compression *until proved otherwise*.
- Recognize that the clinical findings may not be classical. This is elaborated on under the Examination heading. For example, the weakness may be asymmetrical and may be flaccid rather than hypertonic, with both variants being particularly likely during earlier stages of compression.
- Look specifically for confirmatory evidence of cord compression, focusing on symptoms and signs of sensory disturbance producing a 'sensory level' and/or evidence of sphincter involvement with bladder distension, problems with micturition and abnormal anal tone.
- Organize appropriate investigations immediately. This will mean MRI scanning ideally.
- Seek expert neurosurgical advice at the earliest stage.

Associated symptoms

A focused history should involve direct enquiry into additional symptoms associated with the weakness.

Pain

Nerve root lesions may cause pain in the myotome innervated by that root, as illustrated in Table 11.1.

Compression of a peripheral nerve commonly causes dysaesthesiae and even pain in the relevant distribution of that nerve. Fig. 11.2 illustrates the distribution of the peripheral nerves of the hand, for example.

Pain can also be a feature of primary muscle disease. When this occurs, the pain is specifically localized to muscle tissue, often with associated tenderness. Muscle pain or cramping on exercise is a typical symptom in metabolic muscle disease; McArdle's syndrome is the classic example.

Table 11.1 Nerve roots and peripheral nerves in relation to muscles innervated and the movements they subserve

Nerve root(s)	Peripheral nerve(s)	Muscle(s)	Movement to be tested
C5	Axillary	Deltoid	Shoulder abduction
C5,6	Musculocutaneous Radial	Biceps Brachioradialis	Elbow flexion
C7	Radial	Triceps	Elbow extension
C8	Anterior interosseus Ulnar	Long flexors	Finger flexion
T1	Ulnar	Interossei	Finger abduction
T1	Median	Abductor pollicis brevis	Thumb abduction
L1, L2		Iliopsoas	Hip flexion
L5, S1	Sciatic	Gluteus maximus	Hip extension
S1	Sciatic	Hamstrings	Knee flexion
L3, L4	Femoral	Quadriceps	Knee extension
L4, L5	Deep peroneal	Tibialis anterior	Ankle dorsiflexion
S1, S2	Tibial	Gastrocnemius Soleus	Ankle plantarflexion

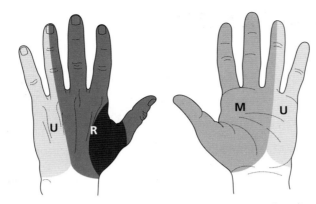

Fig. 11.2 Sensory loss in lesions of the radial (R), ulnar (U) and median (M) nerves as shown. There is overlap in the sensory distribution and the heavily shaded area depicts the maximum sensory loss seen in radial nerve lesions

Fasciculation

Patients may be aware of fasciculation, a phenomenon caused by spontaneous discharge of multiple muscle fibres in a motor unit. Fasciculation is common in motor neurone disease.

Muscle fatigue

The true neurological definition of 'fatigue' refers specifically to 'abnormal failure of strength on repeated muscle contraction'. It is important to differentiate this specific meaning from the more common interpretation of fatigue that is often an articulation of excessive tiredness, which may be due to non-neurological disease as already discussed.

True neurological fatiguability is very suggestive of disease of the neuromuscular junction, particularly myasthenia gravis, and it is worth probing the history specifically for fatiguability of speech, of eye movements or of swallowing during the course of a meal. All of these symptoms are suggestive of myasthenia gravis.

Myotonia

This describes continued involuntary muscle contraction after the subject wishes to cease contraction. The classical example is inability to 'let go' after shaking hands. The most common form of myotonia is myotonic dystrophy, caused by a single gene defect. This condition manifests itself in adulthood and has a number of associated features including frontal baldness, cardiomyopathy, cataracts, diabetes and hypogonadism.

Stroke risk

Assess the patient's stroke risk. Is there a history of hypertension, diabetes, atrial fibrillation, smoking or ischaemic heart disease?

Family history

Always enquire about muscle weakness affecting other family members. Some of the most common inherited disorders are those affecting peripheral nerves and muscle – muscular dystrophies and myotonic dystrophy are examples.

Drug history

Drugs are a major cause of peripheral neuropathy. Cytotoxic agents such as vincristine and cisplatin are examples. Oral corticosteroids are a common cause of proximal muscle weakness, when taken for prolonged periods.

Check also whether the patient is taking potassium-wasting diuretics (e.g. frusemide), as hypokalaemia may be contributing to weakness.

● Examination

Inspection

A focused examination begins with observation of the patient. In particular look for muscle wasting (evidence of LMN pathology) and fasciculation (suggestive of motor neurone disease). Observe the patient's gait: the hypertonic 'scissor' gait of UMN disease is characteristic. Foot drop is easy to detect.

Look for other signs of muscle or neurological disease evident on first inspection: ptosis (myasthenia gravis), frontal balding (myotonic dystrophy), or facial palsy (common in hemisphere strokes).

Power

Table 11.1 on p. 163 lists the movements that should be tested routinely and summarizes the relevant nerve roots, peripheral nerves and muscles that are responsible if power is diminished. Minor degrees of weakness in the lower limbs may be difficult to test on the couch because these muscle groups are naturally very strong. Therefore include other tests of power; ask the patient to:

- stand from a sitting position – this tests hip and knee extensors
- stand on tiptoe – this tests ankle plantarflexion
- walk on the heels – this tests dorsiflexion of the ankles.

Tone and reflexes

The trick in testing tone is to examine the pyramidal tract dominant muscle groups in both the upper and lower limbs. The dominant groups are:

- adduction and internal rotation of the shoulder
- flexion of the elbow
- flexion and pronation of the wrist
- internal rotation at the hip

- extension at the knee
- plantarflexion of the ankle.

Ask the patient to relax and, with a sudden movement, actively extend the elbow and then supinate the wrist in the upper limb. With UMN pathology, characteristic 'clasp-knife' rigidity will be apparent.

The respective movements to assess tone in the lower limb are active external rotation of the hip and active flexion of the knee, respectively (see **Think** below).

Biceps, triceps and supinator reflexes should be tested in the upper limb and knee and ankle reflexes in the legs. Exaggerated reflexes are indicative of a UMN lesion, whereas reflexes will be diminished or absent in LMN pathology.

Plantar reflexes are up-going and down-going with UMN and LMN lesions, respectively.

THINK

How can one effectively assess tone in the lower limbs?

- Because the quadriceps are such powerful muscles it is easy to confuse active resistance from the patient with true rigidity. To obviate this, put your hand behind the patient's knee when they are lying with legs extended on the couch and sharply move their knee upwards. If the patient's heel leaves the bed, this is a good test of hypertonicity.
- A clue to pyramidal tract hypertonicity in the upper limb is *Hoffman's sign*. Hold the patient's middle finger extended at the distal interphalangeal joint and gently flex and then release (flick) their terminal phalanx. If the thumb and other fingers flex, this is suggestive of hypertonicity.
- The clue in the lower limbs is clonus. This should be tested at the ankles (the patient's knees need to be flexed) and at the patella (knees extended).

Coordination

Patients with genuine weakness of the upper or lower limbs may have difficulty in performing the standard tests of coordination such as the 'finger to nose' and 'heel to toe' tests. Coordination may appear to be impaired as a result, even when it is not. Be wary of this; it may lead you to inaccurate localization of the neurological lesion.

Sensory signs

Accompanying sensory signs may help to define the cause of weakness. Fig. 11.2 on p. 164 shows the sensory loss associated with lesions of the radial, ulnar and median nerves. Fig. 11.3

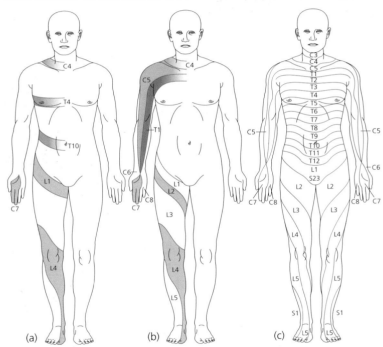

Fig. 11.3 Diagrams to show the dermatomal supply of the upper and lower limbs. (a) Reference dermatomes, (b) dermatomes of the arms and legs, (c) dermatomes on the front of the body. Reproduced with permission from Model D (2006), *Making Sense of Clinical Examination of the Adult Patient* (London: Hodder Arnold)

depicts the dermatomal supply of the upper and lower limbs – weakness due to nerve root pathology may be accompanied by pain and, perhaps, sensory loss in the same dermatome. See also Tables 11.1 (p. 163) and 11.2 (p. 171). The extent of dermatomal sensory loss with a nerve root lesion is very variable, however, and may be minimal or absent despite there being unpleasant pain and/or paraesthesiae. It is important to be aware of the unreliability of objective sensory findings on examination – their absence does not exclude nerve root pathology.

> ## 💡 THINK
>
> *What are the causes of paraparesis?*
> - *Spinal cord compression.* Paraparesis must be considered to be due to spinal cord compression *until proved otherwise*, because of the critical importance of relieving compression quickly.
> - *Guillain–Barré syndrome* (GBS). This is a demyelinating neuropathy that appears to follow an infective illness in a proportion of patients: up to 30 per cent of victims have evidence of a preceding infection with *Campylobacter* and gastrointestinal symptoms to match. The classical presentation of GBS is with an ascending LMN weakness starting from the lower limbs. Pain in muscle groups may be prominent in the early stages, and sensory signs are present though less prominent than the muscular weakness. This is a vital diagnosis to make because weakness may progress to involve the respiratory muscles quite rapidly and respiratory failure may ensue. There are variants of GBS such as the Miller Fisher syndrome, where weakness is often proximal and prominent in the arms in association with ophthalmoplegias of various types and ataxia with nystagmus evident on examination.

- *Anterior spinal artery occlusion*. This can present with symptoms and signs virtually identical to cord compression but, because of the anatomy of the blood supply from this artery, dorsal column sensation is often preserved and this is a useful differentiating feature from cord compression.
- *Transverse myelitis*. An area of demyelination in multiple sclerosis can result in paraparesis.
- *Intramedullary tumours*.

Summary

Table 11.2 is intended as a useful summary of the history and examination findings pertinent to particular localization of the site of a lesion responsible for weakness.

● Investigations

- *Blood tests*. Full blood count and urea and electrolytes are mandatory. In particular, anaemia, evidence of renal impairment and hypokalaemia must be looked for. An elevated creatine kinase points to primary (especially inflammatory) muscle disease.
- *Radiological investigations*. The clinical findings will indicate how to proceed with diagnostic imaging. Computerized tomography of the head with contrast will be indicated for a suspected stroke or intracerebral lesion. MRI will provide far more information if a brain-stem lesion is suspected and is the investigation of choice for suspected cord compression. MRI is also the diagnostic investigation of choice in suspected multiple sclerosis (Fig. 11.4).
- *Nerve conduction studies*. These are usually indicated if a LMN problem is suspected. Both motor and sensory fibre populations can be studied independently. Information is gathered on conduction velocity and the amplitude of individual nerve impulses, and the findings often

Table 11.2 Localization of weakness from history and examination

Site of lesion	Clinical features
Cortical	Lateralized weakness of one or both limbs. Ipsilateral facial weakness and/or homonymous hemianopia may be present. Headache or focal seizures are other potential features
Brain-stem	Many potential associations with lateralized weakness (usually of both limbs), including diplopia, dysarthria, dysphagia, facial sensory loss, vertigo, nystagmus, Horner's syndrome and unsteadiness
Spinal cord	Quadriparesis, paraparesis or hemiparesis may be present depending on the site of the cord pathology. Hemiparesis is a feature of the Brown-Séquard syndrome caused by lesions affecting one half of the spinal cord. Dissociated sensory loss is seen in this syndrome with ipsilateral dorsal column loss (vibration sense and proprioception) and contralateral spinothalamic loss (temperature and pain)

An intrinsic spinal cord tumour can result in upper motor neurone weakness and can also cause an unusual pattern of sensory loss with a band of pain and temperature loss at a certain level with normal sensation above and below. This 'suspended sensory level' is caused by the pattern of recruitment of sensory nerve fibres to the spinothalamic tracts.

The important feature of compressive cord lesions is that symptoms and signs will be related to a 'level' and above this level there will be no abnormality. At the level of the lesion, weakness will be lower motor neurone and below it will be upper motor neurone in type. The signs may be misleading in early stages of spinal cord compression; this, plus the importance of a sensory level together with sphincter disturbance in diagnosing spinal cord compression, has already been emphasized

Compression of the cauda equina results in lower motor neurone weakness with a distribution dependent on the particular nerve roots affected. The distribution of nerves affected can therefore be patchy. Sensory abnormalities are commonly in 'saddle' distribution (roots S2–5) and bladder involvement is frequent with chronic retention of urine being typical |
| Nerve root | Weakness may be associated with sensory loss in the dermatome of the affected root. Muscle pain in the relevant root distribution may be present and associated reflexes will be lost or diminished |
| Ventral horn cell | Fasciculation accompanies the weakness and muscle wasting is prominent. In motor neurone disease there is commonly a mix of upper and lower motor neurone findings because cortical neurones are affected as well as the ventral horn cells |

Continued

Table 11.2 Continued

Site of lesion	Clinical features
Peripheral nerve	Both motor and sensory symptoms and signs are restricted to the distribution of the affected nerve. Weakness is associated with wasting
Neuromuscular junction	Sensory symptoms are absent. Typically weakness of bulbar muscles is prominent in myasthenia gravis and fatiguability is the characteristic association
Muscle	There are no sensory symptoms, and wasting is prominent

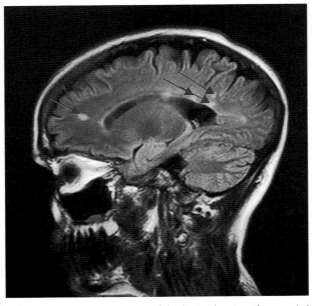

Fig. 11.4 Magnetic resonance image of the brain showing characteristic periventricular white matter lesions (arrowed) in a patient with multiple sclerosis

differentiate between diseases affecting the axon and those affecting the myelin sheath.

- *Electromyography*. EMG detects the electrical activity of muscle fibres and can detect denervation (e.g. in peripheral neuropathy), damage to muscle membranes and other features of primary myopathic diseases. Single-fibre EMG, using a very fine needle, records from one to three muscle fibres and is a useful investigation in myasthenia gravis.

- *Muscle biopsy*. This is useful in categorizing primary muscle disease. It provides a specific diagnosis in some metabolic disorders and in muscular dystrophy as well as in inflammatory muscle disease such as polymyositis.
- *Specific blood tests*:
  - Antibodies to acetylcholine receptors, if positive, confirm the diagnosis of myasthenia gravis. They may be negative in some cases, however, especially in localized forms of the disease such as ocular or bulbar variants.
  - Voltage-gated calcium-channel antibodies are positive in approximately 90 per cent of patients with Eaton–Lambert syndrome, a rare paraneoplastic condition that superficially resembles myasthenia gravis.
  - Rarely, molecular genetic studies are helpful in confirming mitochondrial abnormalities and genetic mutations responsible for some of the hereditary motor-sensory neuropathies (e.g. Charcot–Marie–Tooth disease). These specialist investigations should be undertaken only under the supervision of a neurologist.
- *Lumbar puncture*. This can provide useful information with oligoclonal bands being detected in multiple sclerosis and an elevated protein in cases of Guillain–Barré syndrome.
- *Other investigations*. If an embolic stroke is confirmed then further investigations to quantify stroke risk will be indicated: ECG, echocardiogram, carotid Doppler ultrasound, fasting cholesterol and glucose levels, for example.

12 Abdominal pain

● Introduction

Patients with abdominal pain present to admitting medical teams as well as to surgeons. This is often appropriate because there are a number of non-surgical causes of abdominal pain. However, be alert to the surgical acute abdomen that has been incorrectly referred, and be aware of conditions such as pancreatitis and biliary tract disease where joint medical and surgical management may be beneficial for the patient.

There are two main types of abdominal pain – visceral and peritoneal – both of which can be very severe. Vascular disease and referred pain need to be considered also.

Visceral pain is usually due to disordered motor activity, often as a result of obstruction of a hollow viscus; oesophageal spasm, intestinal, biliary tract and ureteric obstruction are examples. The site of the pain relates to the particular organ involved (see the accompanying classification). It is usually cramping or colicky in nature and the patient often writhes around in an attempt to find a more comfortable position when a spasm of pain occurs. Common causes of visceral pain include obstruction by:

- tumour
- adhesions from earlier surgery

● Classification of abdominal pain

Visceral pain

- *Oesophageal pain* is often in the epigastrium or low central chest.
- *Duodenal pain* is felt in the epigastrium or just to the right of it.
- *Small bowel pain* is poorly localized and is generally felt diffusely in the periumbilical region. Potential causes are:
  - Crohn's disease
  - Enteritis (e.g. due to infective gastroenteritis)
  - Lymphoma and, very rarely, other malignancies.
- *Gall-bladder pain* is most commonly in the right upper quadrant.
- *Pancreatic pain* is felt in the epigastrium but there is often a lot of associated discomfort in the lumbar region of the back. In addition, pancreatitis is a potential cause of generalized abdominal pain and can mimic the peritonism of a ruptured viscus.
- *Ischaemic visceral pain* ('mesenteric angina') is most commonly ischaemia of the bowel due to atherosclerosis and/or embolism of one or other mesenteric artery. Patients are usually elderly and have other evidence of vascular disease or are in atrial fibrillation. Discomfort is more common than severe pain and the diagnosis is often delayed owing to the relative lack of positive findings on abdominal examination, and failure to consider ischaemia as a possible cause early enough. This commonly leads to a poor prognosis.
- *Terminal ileal and colonic pain* is usually sited over the site of pathology. Consider:
  - Carcinoma of the colon
  - Inflammatory bowel disease
  - Irritable bowel syndrome
  - Diverticular disease

– Ischaemic colitis
– Pseudomembranous colitis.

Peritoneal pain

- *Gastric or duodenal perforation*: acid is released into the peritoneum and the pain is excruciating.
- *Gall-bladder rupture*: releases similarly irritant material in the form of bile acids leading again to severe pain.
- *Pancreatitis*: releases pancreatic enzymes, severe pain again results.
- *Small bowel rupture*: uncommon, but can arise from rupture, for example, through a Peyer's patch of typhoid, which is rare in industrialized countries.
- *Colonic rupture*: results in faecal peritonitis. This is often less irritant to the peritoneum and therefore causes less pain.
- *Splenic rupture*: results in bloody peritonitis. It is usually a result of trauma but spontaneous rupture does complicate some splenic pathology.
- *Bloody peritonitis*: results from rupture of major vessels. An aortic aneurysm may rupture through the posterior parietal peritoneum into the peritoneal cavity when signs of generalized peritonitis will follow. Alternatively the blood may remain confined to the retroperitoneal tissues, when the pain will be experienced exclusively in the back.
- *Ruptured ectopic pregnancy*
- *Malignant peritoneal infiltration*: may be from mesothelioma or secondary to carcinoma or lymphoma. The presentation in this context is less acute, occurring over days or weeks.
- *Primary infection*: occurs in primary bacterial peritonitis (usually in association with cirrhosis and this is commonly alcoholic in aetiology) or in tuberculosis. Pain is often not marked in primary infection.

- *'Medical' causes of abdominal pain*: the pain may be severe enough to mimic a surgical 'acute abdomen':
  - Diabetic ketoacidosis – abdominal pain is very common in DKA and is probably caused by a direct effect of the metabolic acidaemia on gut perfusion.
  - Sickle cell crisis – abnormal red cell agglomeration causes pain through gut ischaemia and sometimes splenic infarction.
  - Familial Mediterranean fever is an uncommon inherited condition affecting individuals and families originating from the eastern part of the Mediterranean. It results in recurrent inflammation of serosal surfaces (peritoneum, pleura and pericardium) in association with fever.
  - Acute porphyria (rare).

Referred pain

- *Oesophageal pain* may radiate to the neck or arms.
- *Distal colonic pain* may refer to the lumbar spine.
- *Gall-bladder pain* radiates classically around the lower chest wall to the right infrascapular region.
- *Duodenal ulcer pain* may radiate straight through to the back and this usually indicates penetration of the ulcer into the pancreas.
- *Pain from a subphrenic abscess* irritating the diaphragm may be referred to the shoulder tip.
- *Ureteric colic* has a characteristic radiation from one or other flank around into the lateral abdomen and down to the inguinal region, where it may be felt in the scrotum in men and the labia in women.

- strangulation such as occurs in sigmoid volvulus or strangulated hernia
- strictures (e.g. due to Crohn's disease).

Peritoneal pain originates from the parietal peritoneum. It is caused by perforation of a viscus, pancreatitis, primary peritoneal infection, malignant infiltration or rare types of peritoneal inflammation. Peritoneal pain is exacerbated by even slight movement, especially when caused by perforation of the upper gastrointestinal tract and in pancreatitis when the released fluids are highly irritative. This explains why patients with peritonitis tend to lie perfectly still.

Always consider *vascular pathology* in the patient with abdominal pain. It can be due to rupture of a major vessel (abdominal aortic aneurysm is the classic example) or secondary to ischaemia of the bowel. In women of child-bearing age, always consider ectopic pregnancy as a potential cause as well.

 HAZARD

The spleen enlarges and becomes particularly friable in infectious mononucleosis ('glandular fever'). Patients must be warned to avoid any sort of physical contact, and even over-enthusiastic abdominal examination by medical staff has been reported to result in splenic rupture in the context of glandular fever.

Pain may be *referred* from visceral organs or parietal peritoneum via afferent nerve routes. Pain from a particular site may be referred along dermatome routes that share these afferent nerves and, as a result, experienced at a site distant from its source.

HAZARD

Be wary of thoracic pathology masquerading as an acute abdomen. Pleurisy associated with lower lobe pneumonia or infarction can result in referred pain to one or other upper abdominal quadrant. In addition, 'sympathetic' pleural effusions and lower zone pulmonary consolidation can complicate abdominal pathology in the upper quadrant (the classic example is consolidation secondary to a sub-phrenic abscess). Chest radiograph changes may therefore be either the primary cause of abdominal pain, or secondary to abdominal pathology.

THINK

Are there any features of the pain which indicate that it might be referred?
An area of hyperaesthesia can exist over the referred area and this can be helpful in gall-bladder disease when heightened sensation over the lower border of the scapula supports the diagnosis (Boas' sign).

● History

What does the pain feel like?

Severe, generalized and constant pain that is exacerbated by movement is highly suggestive of peritonitis. *Colicky pain*, in contrast, is likely to be visceral in origin and its characteristics may help to decide which organ is responsible.

- Waves of colicky pain, becoming increasingly severe and then diminishing, are typical of intestinal obstruction. The pain may be generalized or peri-umbilical in site, which suggests small intestinal pathology.
- Longer-lived episodes of pain with less of a crescendo/decrescendo pattern and maximal in the right upper quadrant are suggestive of biliary tract disease.
- The pain of renal colic is often more prolonged, sited in one or other flank and with typical radiation as detailed above.

Where is the pain and does it radiate?

- Pain localized to the right upper quadrant and radiating around to the right infrascapular region is typical of gall-bladder disease.

- Left iliac fossa pain should alert you to pathology in the descending or sigmoid colon (e.g. diverticular disease).
- Pain in the flank radiating around the lateral abdomen and into the scrotum in men or labia in women is highly suggestive of renal colic.
- Pain in the epigastrium points to gastric or, perhaps, pancreatic pathology and the latter is commonly associated with radiation through to the back.
- Right iliac fossa pain should always alert you to the possibility of appendicitis; but if you consider the anatomy of this area it will be clear that pain can also be associated with pathology in a number of other organs – terminal ileum, ascending colon, mesenteric nodes and pelvic organs. All need to be considered.

How did the pain start?

Most causes of abdominal pain start gradually, but perforation of a viscus can cause sudden pain, as can rupture of an abdominal aneurysm.

Are there relieving or exacerbating features?

- Relief of pain by food is a strong pointer to peptic ulceration.
- Exacerbation by food, in contrast, implies gastritis or oesophagitis (in which case, spicy or hot foods may be particularly culpable) or may indicate intestinal obstruction where the pain is exacerbated by the gastro-colic reflex.
- Gastric or duodenal inflammation is often associated with alcohol or NSAID ingestion.
- Oesophageal pain is typically exacerbated by bending or stooping.
- Pain that is aggravated by tension or anxiety is a feature of irritable bowel syndrome.

What is the timing of the pain?

- The pain of duodenal ulceration is typically severe in the early hours of the morning. In addition, the pain may be

periodic with nightly attacks for a few weeks followed by a symptom-free period.
- Diffuse abdominal pain appearing 20 minutes to an hour after meals raises the possibility of mesenteric angina.

Are there risk factors for vascular disease?

If there are, consider the possibility of ischaemic colitis or mesenteric angina.

How long has the pain been present?

- Severe pain persisting for several hours implies viscal perforation, strangulation or intestinal obstruction. Surgical assistance is required.
- Biliary pain becomes progressively more intense with time but can be relieved suddenly with the passage of a stone, leaving a dull, aching sensation in the right upper quadrant. The same thing can happen with renal stones.

Have there been any episodes of diarrhoea?

Diarrhoea might indicate any of the following.

- *Infective gastroenteritis*. This may be due to organisms such as *Salmonella*, *Shigella* or *Campylobacter*. Bloody diarrhoea is also possible with many infective causes.
- *Inflammatory bowel disease*. Bloody diarrhoea is usual in ulcerative colitis.
- *Pseudomembranous colitis*. Consider this in patients who have recently had antibiotics, particularly in hospital.
- *Ischaemic colitis*.

See also Chapter 14.

What is the past medical history?

Important points in the past history of a patient presenting with abdominal pain include:

- previous abdominal surgery, as adhesions may result
- any history of inflammatory bowel disease such as Crohn's disease or ulcerative colitis

- previous episodes of unexplained abdominal pain, which may point to a chronic relapsing aetiology such as Crohn's disease.

Always consider pelvic pathology. Ask about associated symptoms of genitourinary disease such as vaginal discharge. Ask women of child-bearing age about their last menstrual period and the possibility of pregnancy. Previous episodes of pelvic inflammatory disease increase the risk of an ectopic pregnancy.

● Examination

Be systematic in your approach.

How sick is the patient?
- What is the state of hydration?
- Is there haemodynamic compromise? Note the pulse rate, blood pressure, capillary refill time and general appearance of the patient.
- Is there evidence of sepsis, either generalized or localized to the abdomen?

Is this a surgical acute abdomen?
Is an early surgical opinion required? Signs of peritonism should be sought:

- board-like rigidity of the abdomen
- paucity or lack of bowel sounds
- generalized abdominal tenderness.

Is there evidence of intestinal obstruction? Look for:

- visible peristalsis
- abdominal distension
- obstructed ('tinkling') bowel sounds.

Are there localized abnormalities?
- Examine for local tenderness.
- Examine for a palpable mass.

- Is there an enlarged organ? Look specifically for hepatomegaly, splenomegaly, enlargement of the gall bladder and renal masses.

> ### THINK
>
> *What are the characteristics of a renal mass?*
> It is a mass in the lateral abdomen that is bimanually palpable.
>
> - Bilateral renal masses may be due to polycystic kidneys or bilateral hydronephrosis in renal tract obstruction.
> - Bilateral renal masses can be confused with hepatosplenomegaly, but the latter is not bimanually palpable.
> - For the same reason, always sit the patient upright and examine the renal angles. Renal masses will be seen commonly as convex swellings replacing the usual concavity of the renal angles in the flank.
> - As well as polycystic kidneys and hydronephrosis, consider hypernephroma, pyonephrosis, perinephric abscess or haematoma.

- Always examine for femoral, inguinal and peri-umbilical hernia. A strangulated hernia may be accompanied by trophic changes (purplish discolouration and other signs of poor perfusion) in the overlying skin.
- Rectal examination is mandatory. Examine for impacted stool that may be responsible for intestinal obstruction. Alternatively, the rectum may be empty in small or large bowel obstruction from other causes.
- Always examine the right iliac fossa carefully and remember the ancillary signs of appendicitis.

THINK

What are the signs of appendicitis?
- There is tenderness in the right iliac fossa, and tenderness on rectal examination, particularly with pressure to the right side.
- Pressure in the left iliac fossa produces discomfort in the right iliac fossa (Rovsing's sign).
- The patient may be flushed, and the breath is often offensive.
- There may be signs of localized or generalized peritonitis with guarding.

Are there risk factors for ischaemic colitis or mesenteric angina?

Our ageing population makes this diagnosis more common. Consider:

- signs of peripheral or coronary vascular disease
- atrial fibrillation.

Pelvic examination

If this is indicated, ask for a gynaecological review.

● Investigations

Blood tests

- *Full blood count.* Look for anaemia, which may indicate acute blood loss or 'anaemia of chronic disease'.
- *White cell count.* Look for changes suggestive of sepsis.
- *Urea and electrolytes.* Non-specific abnormalities will be seen in anyone who is ill, but there may be specific pointers to renal disease.

- *Liver function tests.* Look for abnormalities of a 'hepatitic' picture or of obstruction, pointing to biliary tract disease. This topic is covered in more detail in Chapter 15.
- *Serum amylase or lipase.* Massive elevation (at least five times normal levels) indicates acute pancreatitis. Less marked elevations are less specific and common in many causes of abdominal pain, particularly intestinal perforation.
- *Markers of infection, inflammation and severe illness.* Look for hypoalbuminaemia (a useful marker of severity in inflammatory bowel disease), elevations of C-reactive protein and ESR.
- *Serum beta-HCG* (pregnancy test). Do this if the patient is of child-bearing age.

Stool culture

This is mandatory in the presence of diarrhoea. Ask particularly for testing for *Clostridium difficile* and its toxin, particularly if the patient has recently taken antibiotics.

Radiographs

Erect and supine abdominal x-rays

- Look for evidence of a perforated viscus with air under the diaphragms (Fig. 12.1).
- Look for intestinal obstruction with characteristic dilated loops of bowel and multiple fluid levels (Fig. 12.2). The haustral pattern may help to differentiate large from small bowel pathology.
- With localized pathology there may be:
  - a dilated, contiguous loop of bowel in cholecystitis
  - a characteristic pattern of bowel dilatation in sigmoid volvulus
  - a classic appearance of toxic megacolon in exacerbation of ulcerative colitis
  - a mucosal pattern suggestive of ischaemic colitis, including 'thumb-printing'.

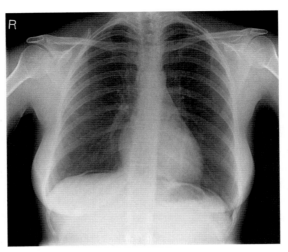

Fig. 12.1 Erect chest x-ray study showing air under both hemidiaphragms in a patient with a perforated viscus

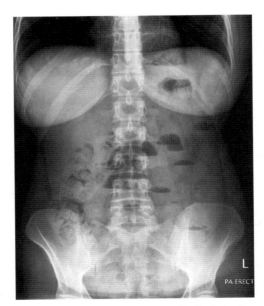

Fig. 12.2 Small bowel obstruction in a patient with Crohn's disease. Note the multiple fluid levels

Chest x-ray

Look for:

- chest pathology manifesting as an 'acute abdomen' (e.g. lower lobe pneumonia)
- pulmonary complications of abdominal pathology (e.g. a left-sided pleural effusion in pancreatitis)
- aspiration pneumonia.

A chest x-ray is often helpful in detecting air below the diaphragms and has the added advantage of being possible with a portable x-ray machine.

Ultrasound

This is particularly useful in investigating potential biliary and renal tract disease. This topic is covered in detail in Chapter 15.

Computerized tomography

This is a vital aid to identifying local pathology as well as detecting free peritoneal fluid.

- CT is often helpful in determining the site and cause of intestinal obstruction. Its usefulness here is enhanced by intravenous contrast.
- It is similarly helpful in determining the nature of abnormal masses and organomegaly.
- It is more reliable than ultrasound in diagnosing pancreatic disease.
- CT is virtually diagnostic in aortic aneurysm rupture.

Sigmoidoscopy

Consider early sigmoidoscopy if exacerbation of inflammatory bowel disease or pseudomembranous colitis is suspected. An urgent gastroenterological review may be required depending on the facilities available because, in these circumstances, the appearances can be characteristic to the experienced observer.

13 Haematemesis and melaena

● Introduction

Haematemesis refers to the vomiting of blood. It encompasses a spectrum of vomitus ranging from bright red, fresh blood at one extreme to old, altered blood, classically described as 'coffee grounds', at the other. Melaena is faeces containing digested blood which has passed through the gut from an origin proximal to the caecum.

Melaena has a typical black, sticky, tarry appearance and a memorably offensive smell. The presence of either fresh haematemesis or melaena indicates that acute bleeding has occurred in the upper gastrointestinal (GI) tract and this is a common cause for presentation to emergency medical services.

> ### THINK
>
> *What are the diagnostic features of a Mallory–Weiss tear?* Typically an episode of fresh haematemesis follows soon after one or more episodes of copious vomiting. This is most common in young men following an alcoholic binge. Upper GI endoscopy is often normal because the oesophageal tear heals quickly, but remember that the bleeding from a tear can be both dramatic and recurrent.

● Classification of haematemesis and melaena

Common causes of acute upper GI bleeding

- Upper GI inflammation, often caused by alcohol or non-steroidal anti-inflammatory drugs (NSAIDS):
  - Reflux oesophagitis
  - Gastritis
  - Duodenitis
- Peptic ulcer disease:
  - Duodenal ulcer – overwhelmingly caused by *Helicobacter pylori* colonization
  - Gastric ulcer (less common than duodenal ulcer)
- Complications of chronic liver disease (from any cause):
  - Oesophageal varices
  - Coagulopathy
- Increased bleeding tendency due to anticoagulant therapy:
  - Warfarin or other coumarins
  - Aspirin
  - Heparin

Less common causes of haematemesis and melaena

- Mallory–Weiss tear of the lower oesophagus. Classically this is a complication of copious vomiting (commonly in association with binge drinking) but occasionally the history of vomiting can be unimpressive.
- Upper GI malignancy:
  - Carcinoma of the oesophagus
  - Carcinoma of the stomach
- Angiodysplasia (arteriovenous malformation of the GI tract)
- Primary bleeding disorder:
  - Thrombocytopenia
  - Clotting factor deficiencies

- Very recent thrombolytic therapy, for example for an acute myocardial infarction
- Nosebleeds – occasionally a large nosebleed may lead to ingestion of enough blood to result in an episode of melaena.

HAZARD

The classical teaching is that acute upper GI bleeding results in melaena while acute lower GI bleeding leads to the passing of red blood per rectum. Note that a really massive life-threatening upper GI bleed may actually result in the passing of red blood per rectum. This is because gut motility may be stimulated so much by the presence of blood that there is no time for melaena to form. Consider this possibility in any shocked patient passing red blood per rectum.

HAZARD

The presence of black stools does not necessarily mean that the patient has melaena. A number of dietary and pharmaceutical agents can colour the stools black. Common examples are oral iron supplements, bismuth salts, liquorice and food containing animal blood such as 'black pudding'. Ask about these if you are not convinced that the stool consists of true melaena (for instance, if the stool consistency is normal and there is no offensive melaena smell).

● History

The likely source of the bleeding can often be ascertained by taking a focused history.

- **Alcohol**. Ask about alcohol intake, recent and habitual. Both acute and chronic alcohol excess can cause upper GI inflammation. An upper GI bleed may be the first presentation of chronic liver disease.
- **Drugs**. Take a detailed drug history including both prescribed and over-the-counter preparations. Ascertain in particular whether the patient has been taking non-steroidal anti-inflammatory drugs (NSAIDs) or oral steroid therapy (both increase the risk of upper GI inflammation and peptic ulceration) or anticoagulant therapy.
- **History of liver disease**. If there is a history of liver disease there is an increased chance of the presence of both oesophageal varices and coagulopathy.
- **Haematemesis as the presenting complaint**. Was blood present in the first vomit or did it appear later? This question helps to determine whether the cause could be a Mallory–Weiss tear of the oesophagus (see **Think** on p. 188).
- **Epigastric pain**. Recent episodes of epigastric pain may indicate peptic ulceration. Classically, the pain of a duodenal ulcer occurs at night and is relieved by eating, whereas pain from a gastric ulcer is said to worsen after eating and this can result in reduced dietary intake and therefore weight loss.
- **Symptoms suggestive of malignancy**. These include insidious onset of weight loss, loss of appetite or dysphagia.
- **Epistaxis**. A recent large nosebleed can occasionally cause melaena.

● Examination

Haemodynamics

Assess haemodynamic status first, with attention to pulse rate, blood pressure, jugular venous pressure, skin pallor or poor peripheral perfusion and prolonged capillary refill time. If there is evidence of haemodynamic compromise (tachycardia, hypotension), resuscitative measures including the insertion of large-bore intravenous (IV) cannulae and IV fluid therapy take precedence over everything else.

⚡ HAZARD

- In previously fit young patients, the pulse rate is a better indicator of volume status than blood pressure. Young adults with healthy hearts maintain their blood pressure for longer in the face of volume loss by means of an increased heart rate. In the context of an upper GI bleed, a raised pulse rate in a younger patient (who looks otherwise stable) is a serious sign of significant volume loss and should prompt immediate large-bore IV cannulation and fluid resuscitation.
- Another sign of continuing blood loss in younger fit patients is the diminishing pulse pressure (difference between systolic and diastolic blood pressure) seen when hypovolaemia is compensated by systemic vasoconstriction. This results in a stable systolic blood pressure but a climbing diastolic blood pressure. The sign is often missed, and this is important because compensatory mechanisms can fail suddenly with a precipitate fall in mean arterial pressure. This compensatory mechanism is either absent or significantly blunted in the elderly and infirm.

Chronic liver disease

Look for evidence of chronic liver disease:

- spider naevi
- palmar erythema
- leuconychia
- ascites

- bruising and bleeding into the skin
- poor nutrition and muscle wasting.

If you find such features, progress to look for evidence of *hepatic encephalopathy* as it indicates the presence of more advanced liver failure, a worse prognosis and a requirement for urgent intervention.

> **THINK**
>
> *What are the clinical features of hepatic encephalopathy?*
> - Confusion or altered consciousness.
> - Asterixis ('liver flap') of the hands.
> - Hepatic fetor is a characteristic sickly sweet smell on the patient's breath.
> - Constructional apraxia is a classical sign and refers to an inability of the patient to copy a five-pointed star drawn by the examining doctor.

Lymphadenopathy

Examine for lymph nodes. Their presence may indicate a malignant process. A palpable node in the left supraclavicular fossa ('Virchow's node') is an indicator of potential malignancy in the upper GI tract or thorax.

Rectal examination

Melaena on your gloved finger corroborates the history. The presence of red blood per rectum may indicate a much larger and potentially life-threatening bleed (see **Hazard** on p. 190).

General abdominal examination

Although it is an important part of the overall assessment of the patient, a general abdominal examination is not usually helpful in determining the precise cause of upper GI bleeding.

● Investigations

Laboratory investigations

The following urgent blood tests should be performed in any patient with evidence of an acute upper GI bleed. In a patient who is haemodynamically compromised, bloods should be sent immediately on presentation and in parallel with resuscitative measures and preliminary history and examination. The detailed history and examination is undertaken when the patient is haemodynamically stable and while the laboratory is processing the urgent tests.

- *Full blood count* – with particular attention to haemoglobin, platelet count and haematocrit.
- *Haemoglobin*. Remember that the haemoglobin level immediately after a bleed may underestimate the degree of blood loss. This is because of subsequent haemodilution: over one or two days following blood loss, fluid moves from the extravascular space into the intravascular space to replenish circulating volume. Natural haemodilution is, of course, potentiated by IV fluid therapy. A repeat haemoglobin after a few hours therefore usually reveals a drop after IV fluid therapy has been administered, even if the patient is stable.
- *Platelet count*. The platelet count often rises above normal after an acute bleed. This is a normal physiological response to bleeding.
- *Haematocrit*. This describes the percentage of blood volume that is composed of red blood cells. As it is a ratio it remains normal immediately after a bleed and only drops with haemodilution as described above.
- *Clotting screen*. Look for a prolonged prothrombin time, particularly in patients with clinical evidence of chronic liver disease. Patients on warfarin will have this expressed as an international normalized ratio (INR). In the context

of acute bleeding, any prolongation of prothrombin time requires urgent correction with agents such as vitamin K and fresh frozen plasma.

- *Blood 'group and hold'*. This is important because it facilitates later cross-matching for transfusion if required. If the patient is shocked, ask the laboratory to cross-match 4 units of blood immediately.
- *Urea and electrolytes*. The serum urea is usually elevated after an acute upper GI bleed as a result of absorption of blood products via the gut.
- *Liver function tests*. Abnormalities suggest acute or chronic liver disease.

CLINICAL TIP

Occasionally, you will be in a situation where possible upper GI bleeding has been reported with no corroboration or first-hand observation by clinical staff. A common example is coffee-ground vomiting reported in an elderly, cognitively impaired patient before arrival in hospital. The description of 'coffee ground' vomitus is often not a reliable indicator of the presence of blood. In this situation there are strategies that help in investigation and management because upper GI endoscopy may pose a risk to a frail patient.

- Test the coffee-ground vomitus (if still available) with a reagent strip for the presence of occult blood.
- Measure the haemoglobin level, with a repeat test the following morning. If the patient is not haemodynamically compromised and the haemoglobin level does not drop, significant blood loss is unlikely and, depending on individual clinical circumstances, further investigation may not be indicated.

Diagnostic investigations

Upper GI endoscopy

In the vast majority of cases of acute upper GI bleeding, this is the only diagnostic test required. Upper GI inflammation, peptic ulceration, oesophageal varices and malignancy can all be confidently diagnosed. In addition, further diagnostic and interventional procedures can be carried out.

Biopsies can be taken for confirmation where a suspected malignant lesion is seen, and for *Helicobacter pylori* testing. The latter can be done either by formal histology or (more commonly) by a rapid urease test. A gastric antral biopsy is placed in a commercially available cartridge in the endoscopy room. A positive result is indicated within hours by a change in colour of the reagent in the cartridge, without the need for further laboratory procedures.

In the case of oesophageal varices, therapeutic intervention to stop bleeding is also possible using techniques such as banding of varices or injection of a sclerosant.

⚡ HAZARD

A second episode of upper GI bleeding, occurring within hours or days of the first, is often referred to as a 're-bleed' and constitutes an emergency as mortality rises steeply once bleeding recurs. This is an indication for urgent out-of-hours gastroenterological and surgical referral.

Recurrent episodes

In some cases no cause for haematemesis or melaena can be identified on upper GI endoscopy. If the patient recovers quickly and there is no recurrence, further investigation may not be indicated. Recurrent episodes will, however, require further investigation and specialist referral.

A detailed description of the investigation of recurrent upper GI bleeding of unknown cause is beyond the scope of this text, but possible investigations in this situation include:

- mesenteric angiogram, looking for arteriovenous malformations
- video capsule endoscopy, to visualize the small bowel lumen distal to the range of a standard endoscope
- double-balloon enteroscopy – a technique allowing excellent visualization of the entire small bowel lumen.

14 Diarrhoea and vomiting

● Introduction

The differential diagnosis of vomiting is broad and so is that of diarrhoea. On the other hand, when vomiting and diarrhoea are both part of the clinical presentation then the potential aetiology is less varied and an infective cause is most likely. The accompanying classification has further details.

A second point to make is the importance of bleeding as part of the presenting symptomatology. Haematemesis and melaena are the subject of Chapter 13 and will not be discussed here, but 'bloody diarrhoea' is an important clinical presentation, which has a clear differential diagnosis and it is discussed below.

Our daily intake of food and liquid, combined with gastric and intestinal secretions, results in a volume load of approximately 7 litres for the small intestine. By the time intestinal contents have reached the terminal ileum this volume has been reduced to approximately 1.5 litres, illustrating the role played by the small intestine in fluid absorption and explaining why the hallmark of small bowel pathology is large-volume diarrhoea.

'Diarrhoea is difficult to define but easy to appreciate if you have it!' This humorous definition is close to the truth, but a more scientific definition is necessary as well. A careful history is

● Classification of diarrhoea and vomiting

Vomiting alone

- Obstructing lesions:
  - Malignant disease of the upper gastrointestinal tract
  - Benign tumours – leiomyoma of the stomach is an example
  - Pyloric stenosis, commonly the result of chronic peptic ulceration
  - Small intestinal obstruction, where the classical appearance is of foul, 'faeculent' vomiting of partially digested food
- Infections:
  - Food or drink infected with organisms that produce exotoxins (*Staphylococcus* is a typical example) commonly produces gastroenteritis where vomiting is exclusive or far more pronounced than diarrhoea
  - Norovirus infection
  - Viral hepatitis
- Sepsis:
  - Vomiting is a common non-specific symptom of generalized sepsis
  - Cholecystitis
  - Urinary tract infection
- Metabolic causes:
  - Uraemia
  - Hepatic failure
  - Hypercalcaemia (although nausea is a more common symptom than actual vomiting in this context)
- Endocrinological disease:
  - Diabetic keto-acidosis – vomiting is very common
  - Uncommonly, in thyrotoxicosis and Addison's disease

- Neurological conditions:
  - Raised intracranial pressure
  - Labyrinthine pathology commonly results in severe nausea and vomiting
  - Brain-stem pathology also – refer to Chapter 8
- Pregnancy
- Drugs (common examples):
  - Illicit drugs (though marijuana has been used as an antiemetic)
  - Alcohol excess
  - Antibiotics
  - Chemotherapeutic agents
  - Antidepressants
  - Analgesics, especially opiates
- Psychiatric conditions – especially eating disorders, anorexia nervosa and bulimia
- Severe constipation – particularly in elderly patients

Diarrhoea alone

- Infections (see Table 14.1):
  - Viral gastroenteritis – many different viruses can be responsible and these are often highly contagious
  - Bacterial: *Salmonella*, *Shigella*, *Vibrio cholerae*, *Yersinia*, *Campylobacter*, *Escherichia coli*
  - Protozoa – especially *Giardia lamblia*
  - Amoebae – especially *Entamoeba histolytica*
- Neoplastic disease:
  - Colonic carcinoma
  - Villous adenoma of the rectum – the diarrhoea is often marked and results in the characteristic combination of hypokalaemia and acidosis due to loss of potassium and bicarbonate, respectively
  - Small bowel lymphoma – uncommon but associated with untreated chronic coeliac disease

- Irritable bowel syndrome – pain or diarrhoea (and occasionally constipation) may predominate
- Inflammatory bowel disease:
  - Crohn's disease can affect any part of the bowel from mouth to anus
  - Ulcerative colitis is a colonic and rectal disease
  - Both are associated with bloody diarrhoea
- Endocrinological:
  - Thyrotoxicosis
  - Addison's disease may have diarrhoea as well as abdominal discomfort as part of its presenting symptomatology
  - Zollinger–Ellison syndrome (very rare) – the excessive amounts of gastrin produced by the gastrinoma(s) result in diarrhoea as well as peptic ulceration in unusual sites
- Malabsorption:
  - Coeliac disease
  - Giardiasis (has been mentioned above)
  - Tropical sprue – mainly confined to the tropics within 30 degrees north or south of the equator, consider in people who have visited such regions for more than a month
  - Intestinal bacterial overgrowth – can occur following intestinal surgery and in chronic liver disease, chronic pancreatitis and immunodeficiency among other causes
  - Tape-worm infestation
  - Terminal ileitis – disruption of bile acid reabsorption results in an irritative colonic diarrhoea
  - Disaccharidase deficiency – may follow a severe bout of diarrhoea (simple lactose intolerance is more common)
- Drugs:
  - Antibiotics

- Antacids, particularly proton pump inhibitors
- Non-steroidal anti-inflammatory drugs
- Laxatives
- 'Overflow diarrhoea' in severely constipated elderly patients

Bloody diarrhoea

This is an important symptom. Consider especially:
- Inflammatory bowel disease
- Infections, particularly *Salmonella*, *Shigella*, amoebic dysentery, *Campylobacter* (sometimes)
- Ischaemic colitis – particularly in elderly patients with vascular disease risk factors

Diarrhoea and vomiting combined

Most of the diagnoses already mentioned can be associated with a combination of diarrhoea and vomiting with a preponderance of one or the other. However, when diarrhoea and vomiting appear equally prominent, gastroenteritis due to infective agents is easily the most likely cause.

required in order to be certain that diarrhoea is genuinely present. Increased frequency of watery stools is generally regarded as evidence of diarrhoea.

The nature of the diarrhoea is important in diagnosis, as follows.

- Frequent passage of small amounts of stool is common in proctitis and other rectal pathology.
- Large volumes of diarrhoea most commonly imply small bowel pathology.
- A history of bloody diarrhoea is highly suggestive of colonic pathology.
- Copious, bulky stools that are foul-smelling and difficult to flush away are characteristic of malabsorption.

Table 14.1 Intestinal infections, including salient points of enquiry in patients presenting with diarrhoea

Site of infection	Infectious agent	Predisposing cause/features
Small bowel	Cholera	Foreign travel
	Enterotoxigenic E. coli	Infected meat
		Common and associated with vomiting
	Viruses (rotavirus, norovirus, small round virus)	Vomiting associated
	Bacteria producing toxins	*Staphylococcus aureus*: symptoms a few hours after ingestion of contaminated material
		Bacillus cereus: classically associated with contaminated rice
Colon	*Campylobacter*	Inadequately-cooked chicken and rice
	Shigella and *Salmonella*	Classic cause of dysentery
		Cause bloody diarrhoea
	Enterohaemorrhagic E. coli	May be associated with haemolytic uraemic syndrome and thrombotic thrombocytopenic purpura
	Clostridium difficile	Toxin-producing, associated with antibiotic therapy
		Diarrhoea is often very foul-smelling
	Amoebiasis	Can be contracted in UK and other Western countries, so an important consideration on acute medical 'intake'

CLINICAL TIP

Always consider *hypercalcaemia* as a potential cause of unexplained vomiting. If hypercalcaemia is responsible, the underlying pathology is usually either malignancy or hyperparathyroidism.

● History

Is there vomiting, diarrhoea or both?
If there are both, then which is the dominant symptom? The preceding classification will prove useful in narrowing the differential diagnosis.

When did the symptoms start and are there precipitating factors?
Potentially contaminated food or water is an obvious culprit. Question also for drug use:

- Has there been a recent prescription of antibiotics?
- Are non-steroidal anti-inflammatory drugs (NSAIDs) taken regularly?

Both can cause diarrhoea.

- Similarly, is there any medication that might be associated with vomiting?

Is there a previous history of bowel problems?
Ask about:

- recurrent dyspepsia and symptoms suggestive of peptic ulceration
- previous episodes of diarrhoea with mucus and/or blood associated (inflammatory bowel disease is a potential diagnosis)
- inflammatory bowel disease (a colonic neoplasm may complicate longstanding ulcerative colitis)
- previous bowel surgery
- abdominal irradiation ('radiation colitis' can present with bloody diarrhoea).

What is the duration of symptoms?

- Long-standing diarrhoea, often periodic and alternating with periods of constipation in a person who is clearly not ill, suggests irritable bowel syndrome (IBS).
- On the other hand, longstanding symptoms with weight loss, perhaps anaemia and additional symptoms may imply malabsorption.

- Recurrent diarrhoea with general symptoms of weight loss, abdominal pain and systemic upset is compatible with inflammatory bowel disease (IBD).

What is the nature of the diarrhoea?

Particular features include:

- malabsorption – bulky, offensive motions that are difficult to flush away
- large-volume diarrhoea – small bowel aetiology
- bloody diarrhoea – colonic pathology
- nocturnal diarrhoea – a good indicator of organic pathology, but uncommon in IBS.

Ask about the vomiting

- Vomiting occurring shortly after eating suggests an obstructive lesion.
- Faeculent vomiting suggests small-intestinal obstruction.

Are there associated symptoms?

- Weight loss will alert you to serious pathology.
- Joint problems can be associated with IBD.
- Skin rashes occur with IBD and coeliac disease (see below under Examination).

Is there other relevant pathology?

For example, sudden onset of pain with diarrhoea (that may be bloody) in an elderly arteriopath will alert you to the possibility of ischaemic colitis. Is HIV a possibility? Consider HIV-related bowel infections, for example Cytomegalovirus and Cryptosporidiosis.

● Examination

Physiological instability

As always, focus your examination and commence with an assessment of how unwell the patient is. These general observations are just as important as the localized abdominal findings.

Haemodynamics

Check:

- pulse rate
- peripheral perfusion, including capillary refill time
- blood pressure
- mean arterial pressure as an arbiter of tissue perfusion (see **Think** below).

Fluid balance

- Assess the central venous pressure and decide whether the patient is hypovolaemic.
- The presence of peripheral oedema indicates salt and water overload.
- If oedema is present with a low venous pressure, this is highly suggestive of hypoproteinaemia – a feature of protein-losing enteropathy and a marker of severity in IBD.

Sepsis

Check for:

- hyperthermia
- hypothermia
- signs of septic shock, including evidence of organ hypoperfusion (mental confusion, oliguria).

THINK

How does one calculate mean arterial pressure, and why is this important?

The mean arterial pressure (MAP) is an important arbiter of tissue perfusion. It is easily calculated: measure the pulse pressure (systolic BP minus diastolic BP), divide this by 3, and add the result to the diastolic blood pressure. This calculation takes into account the differential times occupied by systole and diastole during the cardiac cycle in their contribution to mean arterial blood pressure. To put things in a clinical perspective, a MAP of less than 65 mmHg is diagnostic of a shock state.

Examine for systemic illness

- **Jaundice**. Deep jaundice is suggestive of biliary tract obstruction. Look for ancillary evidence of this diagnosis with gall-bladder distension (Courvoisier's sign), pale stools and dark urine.
- **Lymphadenopathy**. Take care to examine for a node in the left supraclavicular area (Virchow's node). Hard lymphadenopathy in this site is often associated with upper GI malignancy.
- **Skin rashes**. Dermatitis herpetiformis is a characteristic association of coeliac disease (see Chapter 18). Erythema nodosum is an (uncommon) accompaniment of IBD.
- **Joint pathology**. Joint swelling and arthralgia are associated with IBD.

Systematic abdominal examination

- **Pain**. Enquire about local or generalized abdominal pain and respect this as you proceed with your examination.
- **Guarding**. Is there localized or generalized guarding, suggesting peritonism and peritonitis, respectively?
- **Abnormal masses**. Examine for local masses and organomegaly. Also consider the possibility of faecal loading as this is a common cause of 'overflow' diarrhoea (and sometimes vomiting) in the elderly.
- **Gastric outflow obstruction**. There may be fullness and discomfort in the epigastrium and a succussion splash may be present. Grip the patient's pelvis and shake their abdomen from side to side with your stethoscope placed over the epigastrium. A characteristic 'splash' will be heard.
- **Intestinal obstruction**. Examine for:
  - abdominal distension
  - visible peristalsis
  - obstructed ('tinkling') bowel sounds.

Perineum and rectal examination

- **Perineum**. Look for skin tags, fissures or fistulae suggestive of Crohn's disease.
- **Rectum**. Search for a possible mass, and inspect any faeces on the glove for melaena or frank blood.

● Investigations

Blood tests

Haematology

- *Anaemia*. This may be acute if there is heavy GI bleeding, but its presence is more likely to indicate chronic blood loss, malabsorption or inadequately controlled IBD.
- *MCV, MCH and blood film*. Microcytic, hypochromic changes are most likely due to iron deficiency and commonly indicate chronic blood loss. Importantly, they may be seen as the only abnormality in coeliac disease, especially when this presents in later life. Macrocytosis points to vitamin B_{12} and/or folic acid deficiency and is also seen in chronic alcohol abuse.
- *White cell count*. Significant elevation of white cell count (>15 000) should alert you to sepsis, but leucopaenia is also a marker for sepsis and suggests severe sepsis when it is present in association with other features of infection.

Biochemistry

- *Urea and electrolytes*. These should be checked routinely. Severe illness, with or without dehydration, will result in impaired renal function and a variety of electrolyte abnormalities can accompany diarrhoea and vomiting.
  - Severe vomiting results in loss of hydrochloric acid in gastric secretions and a profound hypochloraemic alkalosis may ensue.
  - At the *other end*, severe colonic diarrhoea results in loss of bicarbonate and potassium because both ions are

abundant in colonic contents. The hypokalaemic acidosis that results is characteristic and the only other situation where this combination is encountered is in renal tubular acidosis.

Blood cultures

Any suggestion of sepsis mandates immediate blood cultures.

Inflammatory markers

- *C-reactive protein* (CRP). Elevation of CRP above 45 mg/L is a marker of severity in IBD and is especially so in ulcerative colitis.
- *Serum proteins*. A serum albumin of <30 g/L is a marker of severity in IBD. This is because albumin loss is proportional to the extent of bowel involvement in IBD. It follows that hypoalbuminaemia is particularly worrying in acute ulcerative colitis or colonic Crohn's disease.

 HAZARD

The following features are markers of severity in an exacerbation of *ulcerative colitis*:
- bowels open >10 times in first 24 h
- pulse rate >100/minute
- temperature >38°C
- serum albumin <30 g/L
- CRP >45 mg/L
- abdominal radiographic findings of toxic megacolon, mucosal islands, or dilated small bowel loops.

Tests for malabsorption

Check serum for:

- calcium
- proteins
- B_{12} and red cell folic acid (serum folic acid is not a reliable marker of chronic deficiency)

- iron, ferritin and transferrin (coeliac disease may present with isolated iron-deficiency anaemia)
- transglutaminase antibodies.

The last are more than 90 per cent sensitive for coeliac disease, but complete exclusion of this diagnosis can be achieved only through negative histological findings on duodenal biopsy.

Endocrinological tests
It may be necessary to perform thyroid function tests, a serum cortisol and perhaps perform a synacthen test to exclude Addison's disease.

Serology
Investigate unusual infections (e.g. *Yersinia* colitis) with specific antibody assays.

Stool examination
If diarrhoea is present, send faeces to the laboratory for:

- bacterial culture
- microscopy for ova, cysts and parasites
- *Clostridium difficile* culture and toxin.

Radiology
- *Erect chest x-ray*. This should include the hemidiaphragms in order to exclude air under the diaphragms indicative of viscal perforation.
- *Supine abdominal x-ray*. This is important in diagnosing intestinal obstruction and faecal impaction. It is also vital in detecting toxic colonic dilatation and other bad prognostic radiographic signs of IBD (see **Hazard** above).
- *Ultrasound of the abdomen*. This is indicated particularly in the presence of jaundice. See Chapter 15 for further details.
- *Computerized tomography*. This is indicated particularly if an obstructive or malignant cause is possible.

- *Sigmoidoscopy and colonoscopy.* A specialist referral will be required and should be sought in cases of diarrhoea persisting for more than two weeks (see **Clinical tip** and **Hazards** below).
- *Upper GI endoscopy.* This will investigate upper GI pathologies of ulceration, malignancy and gastric outflow tract obstruction. Duodenal biopsies should be taken to investigate the possibility of coeliac disease.

CLINICAL TIP

Sigmoidoscopy provides useful diagnostic information.

- Inflamed rectal mucosa can be a feature of any cause of severe diarrhoea.
- Normal rectal mucosa usually excludes active ulcerative colitis unless topical steroids have been administered.
- Some rectal appearances are fairly specific: contact bleeding in IBD, ulceration and the typical pseudomembrane of pseudomembranous colitis.

HAZARD

Rectal biopsies should be taken *below the peritoneal reflection* (i.e. within 10 cm of the anal margin) to minimize the risk of perforation and peritonitis.

HAZARD

A supine abdominal film should be taken *before* sigmoidoscopy, because introduction of air during the procedure can result in a subsequent x-ray resembling toxic dilatation.

15 Jaundice

Introduction

Jaundice is an important symptom or sign with many potentially serious, even life-threatening, causes – so achieving a prompt and accurate diagnosis is vital. When jaundice is the presenting problem, the first diagnostic question to answer is whether the cause is obstruction of the common bile duct. This may well require an interventional procedure as distinct from other causes requiring non-interventional treatment. When this fundamental question has been addressed, further assessment should aim to determine the precise cause.

> ### ⚡ HAZARD
> The common textbook classification of jaundice is into pre-hepatic, intra-hepatic (or hepatocellular) and post-hepatic (obstructive or cholestatic) causes. While helpful in listing causes of jaundice, this classification has drawbacks in clinical practice. The aetiology of jaundice does not always fall neatly into one of these groups; for example, elements of hepatocellular and cholestatic jaundice often coexist.

● Classification of jaundice

Common causes of jaundice in acute medicine:
- Mechanical common bile duct (CBD) obstruction due to:
  - Gallstone impaction
  - Malignancy – for example, carcinoma of the head of the pancreas, cholangiocarcinoma or lymphadenopathy at the porta hepatis due to lymphoma
- Advanced cirrhosis due to:
  - Alcoholic liver disease – by far the most common cause of cirrhosis in industrialized countries
  - Less common causes such as chronic hepatitis B or C infection, haemochromatosis, α_1-antitrypsin deficiency, Wilson's disease
- Acute hepatitis due to:
  - Persistent alcohol excess (a common cause)
  - Viral infection – the most common viruses causing acute hepatitis are hepatitis A and B; others include Epstein–Barr virus (EBV) and cytomegalovirus (CMV)
  - Drug toxicity – includes paracetamol overdose. (There are many drugs with the potential to cause hepatitis when used in normal therapeutic doses. A full list is beyond the scope of this text, but well-known examples include anaesthetic agents such as halothane and antituberculous agents such as isoniazid.)
  - Autoimmune hepatitis – a much less common cause of hepatitis

Less common causes of jaundice presenting acutely
- Haemolysis is classically described as a 'pre-hepatic' cause of jaundice and can be subdivided into:
  - Extravascular haemolysis – this is commoner and may be due to red cell defects, haemoglobinopathies or autoimmune conditions, or may be drug-induced

- Intravascular haemolysis – can be the result of mechanical causes such as prosthetic heart valves or be due to infection (for example malaria) or auto-immune disease
- Intrahepatic cholestasis – may be drug-induced or have an unusual aetiology, for example, primary biliary cirrhosis (PBC), sclerosing cholangitis or pregnancy
- Unusual or rare infections – examples include leptospirosis and yellow fever.

CLINICAL TIP

Patients presenting to hospital with haemolysis are more likely to present with symptoms of anaemia rather than complaining predominantly of jaundice. Moreover, jaundice secondary to haemolysis is usually mild in comparison with the other causes of jaundice discussed here.

● History

A careful history is fundamental in making the diagnosis in a jaundiced patient. Ask in particular about the following.

- **Country of origin, recent travel and periods of residence abroad**. Hepatitis B is common in South East Asia, Africa and the Middle East, and patients born in these areas have a higher incidence of chronic hepatitis B infection. Recent travel may raise the possibility of hepatitis A (particularly in areas with poor sanitation), yellow fever or malaria, depending upon the countries visited.
- **Duration and onset**. As a guideline, remember that the incubation period for hepatitis A is 2–6 weeks, and for hepatitis B it is 2–6 months. Insidious onset of jaundice over several weeks increases the likelihood of a malignant cause.

- **Abdominal pain**. Colicky right upper quadrant pain is a symptom of acute biliary obstruction and may indicate common bile duct (CBD) obstruction by a gallstone. More constant upper abdominal or right upper quadrant pain with an enlarged liver may be due to liver capsule pain caused by acute liver enlargement.
- **Alcohol intake**. An accurate alcohol history is important and not always easy to elicit as patients often attempt to conceal the extent of their intake.

> **THINK**
>
> *How can one elicit a more accurate alcohol history in an evasive patient?*
> Phrasing the question in different ways can help in clarifying the situation if you think the patient is being evasive. For example, find out what they drink and then ask how often they buy it.

- **Colour of urine and faeces**. Dark urine and pale faeces are classically described as indicative of obstructive or cholestatic jaundice, but the urine can also be dark in hepatocellular jaundice.
- **Consumption of shellfish**. If this has occurred in the preceding 2–6 weeks, hepatitis A infection is possible.
- **Exposure to other jaundiced individuals**. This raises the possibility of an infective cause, such as hepatitis A.
- **Associated symptoms**. Insidious weight loss may indicate malignancy. The prodrome of hepatitis B before jaundice appears often includes fever, joint pains and a rash. Interestingly, smokers with hepatitis A classically lose their taste for cigarettes during the prodrome.
- **Fever and rigors**. Symptoms suggestive of acute sepsis in the jaundiced patient should prompt consideration of a diagnosis of acute cholangitis. This is a medical emergency.

- **Sexual history**. The risk of hepatitis B infection is increased in sex workers and in men who have sex with men.
- **Drug history**. Take a detailed drug history including prescribed drugs, over-the-counter medications (especially paracetamol), recreational drug use (and always enquire about the route of administration) and other preparations such as Chinese herbal remedies. Acute liver failure can be associated with all of these classes of drugs.
- **History of intravenous drug use and tattoos**. Intravenous drug use increases the risk of hepatitis B and C infection. The presence of tattoos is associated with an increased risk of hepatitis C.
- **History of blood transfusion**. Hepatitis C virus (HCV) was described in 1988 and reliable testing of blood products for HCV was introduced between 1990 and 1992 in many developed countries. A history of blood or blood product transfusion before 1992 (or more recently in developing countries) should raise suspicion of possible HCV infection.

● Examination

There are various examination clues that assist in narrowing the differential diagnosis in a jaundiced patient. Look first for **evidence of chronic liver disease**:

- spider naevi
- palmar erythema
- leuconychia
- ascites
- bruising and bleeding into the skin
- poor nutrition and muscle wasting.

If you find such features, progress to look for the following.

- **Hepatic encephalopathy**. This indicates the presence of more advanced liver failure with a worse prognosis, and requires urgent intervention.

THINK

What are the clinical features of hepatic encephalopathy?

- Confusion or altered consciousness.
- Asterixis ('liver flap') of the hands.
- Hepatic fetor is a characteristic sickly sweet smell on the patient's breath.
- Constructional apraxia is a classical sign and refers to an inability of the patient to copy a five-pointed star drawn by the examining doctor.

- **Signs of gastrointestinal bleeding**, including melaena on rectal examination.
- **Tattoos and needle track marks**. There is an increased possibility of HCV infection.
- **Lymphadenopathy**. This may indicate advanced malignancy.
- **Fever**, which may indicate an acute infective cause (see **Hazard** below).

HAZARD

Fever, rigors and right upper quadrant pain in a jaundiced patient may indicate *acute cholangitis*. This is a medical emergency requiring prompt investigation and treatment with intravenous fluids and antibiotics.

- **Hepatomegaly**. The liver in established cirrhosis is usually smaller than normal. Therefore, hepatomegaly tends to indicate either a more acute inflammatory cause (e.g. acute hepatitis) or that the liver is infiltrated with something causing enlargement, classically malignant metastases. An enlarged liver infiltrated with metastases will often feel irregular or knobbly compared with the enlarged liver of acute hepatitis, which has a smooth edge.

- **Splenomegaly**. This may indicate established portal hypertension due to cirrhosis, particularly if signs of chronic liver disease are present. Less marked enlargement of the spleen is also seen in acute viral hepatitis.
- **Abdominal pain or tenderness**. Causes of upper abdominal or right upper quadrant pain in the jaundiced patient include an acutely enlarged liver (caused by hepatic capsular distension) and an acutely inflamed gall bladder (as in acute cholangitis; see **Hazard** above).

● Investigations

Laboratory investigations

Patients presenting for the first time with jaundice will require a number of urgent blood tests, both to investigate the aetiology and to establish the degree of liver dysfunction.

- *Full blood count*. A raised white cell count may indicate infection, thrombocytopenia may suggest chronic liver disease, and anaemia may point to GI bleeding in chronic liver disease.
- *Urea, electrolytes and blood sugar*. Electrolyte abnormalities are common in chronic liver disease and can precipitate clinical deterioration. Exclude hyponatraemia, hypokalaemia and hypoglycaemia in particular because they all demand urgent correction.
- *Clotting screen*. A prolonged prothrombin time (PT) is a significant finding. It indicates poor liver synthetic function of clotting factors and requires treatment with vitamin K or fresh frozen plasma, or both.
- *Liver function tests*. Most laboratories will provide estimation of:
  - serum albumin
  - a transaminase, either alanine aminotransferase (ALT) or aspartate transaminase (AST)
  - alkaline phosphatase (ALP)

- gamma glutamyltransferase (GGT)
- serum bilirubin.

The results and particularly the degree of elevation of some of these enzymes may help to determine the cause of jaundice (see **Think** below).

- A low serum albumin is common in chronic liver disease due to reduced albumin synthesis.
- A raised GGT is a non-specific finding (common in heavy alcohol drinkers, for example), which is not usually helpful in investigating the precise cause of jaundice.
- The serum bilirubin will always be elevated in a jaundiced patient, usually with a rise in both conjugated and unconjugated bilirubin (see **Think** below).
- Normal liver enzyme levels in a jaundiced patient are suggestive of a 'pre-hepatic' cause such as haemolysis.

THINK

How does the pattern of liver enzyme elevation assist in determining the cause of jaundice?
As a broad generalization, acute hepatitis causes a greater proportionate rise in transaminases (ALT and AST) than ALP; while obstructive jaundice secondary to biliary tract obstruction is the converse, with a greater proportionate rise in ALP compared with transaminases. This is because AST and ALT are produced by the hepatocytes whereas ALP originates from the biliary epithelium.

THINK

Do the relative levels of conjugated and unconjugated bilirubin help in narrowing the differential diagnosis?
To some extent, yes. Obstructive and cholestatic jaundice tend to lead to a more marked rise in serum

conjugated bilirubin, which is water-soluble and then appears in the urine giving a dark colour. Conversely, jaundice from hepatocellular disease such as acute hepatitis tends to cause a greater rise in unconjugated bilirubin because of impaired hepatocellular function. Haemolysis causing jaundice will result in an unconjugated hyperbilirubinaemia simply owing to increased production of bilirubin as there is no defect in conjugation by hepatocytes.

- *Serum paracetamol level*. This should be undertaken if there is any suggestion of paracetamol overdose. Note, however, that the PT gives more accurate prognostic information in this situation.
- *Serology for hepatitis A, B and C viruses, Epstein–Barr virus and cytomegalovirus.*

More specialized blood tests

Tests for rarer causes of liver disease should be requested non-urgently after specialist advice has been sought and mechanical bile duct obstruction ruled out. These might include:

- serum iron, transferrin and ferritin levels to investigate for haemochromatosis
- alpha-1 antitrypsin levels for cirrhosis due to α_1-AT deficiency
- caeruloplasmin levels for Wilson's disease
- antimitochondrial antibodies, which are positive in primary biliary cirrhosis
- anti-smooth muscle and liver/kidney microsomal antibodies to investigate autoimmune hepatitis.

If a diagnosis of haemochromatosis is likely, further genetic testing for the C282Y mutation of the haemochromatosis gene (known as the HFE gene) is indicated.

Radiological investigations

As stated in the introduction to this chapter, the first diagnostic question to answer is whether jaundice is due to obstruction of the common bile duct. Obstructive causes require intervention with a procedure, as distinct from non-obstructive causes. The available imaging modalities are discussed below.

Ultrasound of the upper abdomen

The quickest and simplest way to determine whether mechanical bile duct obstruction is present is by ultrasound. Bile duct dilation is usually clearly visible and gallstones may also be identified. Note that not all gallstones are detected by ultrasound because gas in the duodenum may obscure them from view.

If bile duct dilation is present, further imaging will be required to determine the precise cause and to plan intervention.

Ultrasound can also reliably pick up cirrhosis and liver metastases, but may not provide good imaging of the pancreas – for which CT is superior.

Endoscopic ultrasound

Ultrasound can also be performed from within the duodenum during an upper GI endoscopy. This has the advantage of eliminating the problem of bowel gas obscuring the view. Gallstones and small pancreatic tumours can be better visualized than with conventional ultrasound or CT. The technique has the disadvantages of being invasive and only available in units with specially trained gastroenterologists, but it may become more widely available in the future.

Computerized tomography of the abdomen

CT will pick up bile duct dilation (Fig. 15.1) and is better than ultrasound for imaging liver architecture and the other abdominal organs. However, CT has drawbacks and so should

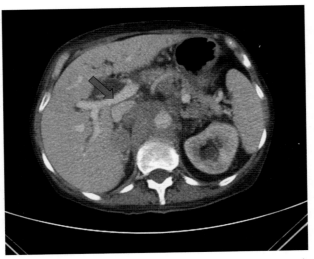

Fig. 15.1 Computerized tomography of the abdomen with contrast, showing grossly dilated bile ducts (arrowed) caused in this case by obstructing lymphadenopathy at the porta hepatis

not be the investigation of choice if obstructive jaundice is thought to be due to gallstones.

- Abdominal CT entails significant radiation exposure.
- It is not good at imaging gallstones as it only picks up those that are calcified.
- Small pancreatic tumours may also be missed.
- Intravenous contrast is required and this poses a risk of renal impairment in sick patients who are poorly hydrated or who have pre-existing renal impairment.

Endoscopic retrograde cholangiopancreatography

ERCP is the most sensitive and specific way to investigate and treat bile duct obstruction, particularly if gallstone obstruction is suspected. The patient undergoes an upper GI endoscopy and the operator inserts a catheter into the common bile duct and injects a radiopaque dye. Obstruction due to gallstones or tumour can be diagnosed and often relieved by removal of a stone or stenting of an obstructing lesion during the procedure. ERCP has the advantage of allowing intervention at the time of the procedure (e.g. sphincterotomy of the ampulla of Vater) to treat the cause of obstructive jaundice. The procedure is invasive, however, and carries risks of postoperative pancreatitis, cholangitis and bleeding.

Magnetic resonance cholangiopancreatography

MRCP is a non-invasive alternative to ERCP. It also has the advantages of not involving radiation and not requiring injection of intravenous contrast. It is sensitive and specific in the investigation of obstructive jaundice and gives the same diagnostic information as that provided by ERCP. The main drawbacks are that very small lesions and gallstones (under 4 mm) may be missed, and intervention is not possible (many patients will go on to require ERCP subsequently). It is also expensive.

CLINICAL TIP

The initial investigations in a jaundiced patient should include the urgent blood tests listed above and ultrasound examination of the upper abdomen. If bile duct obstruction is present, we would argue that the next steps should be urgent gastroenterological review with a view to ERCP or MRCP. If cirrhosis is revealed, further blood tests will be required to investigate the cause. If blood test results suggest acute hepatitis, additional laboratory tests will be required to determine the cause.

16 The patient with a fever

● Introduction

The most common cause of a fever is a self-limiting viral illness. Most patients presenting with a fever to emergency medical services will have an infective cause that is readily identifiable after history, examination and some simple first-line investigations. A minority of pyrexial patients will present a greater diagnostic challenge, usually because of a prolonged fever despite treatment for a presumed cause.

> **THINK**
>
> What is the definition of a 'pyrexia of unknown origin'? PUO is a fever that has persisted for more than three weeks despite extensive investigation and treatment for any suspected cause.

In your diagnostic approach consider first the context in which the fever has arisen. Patient demographics, geographical location, immune status, lifestyle, occupation, hobbies and history of travel may all have a substantial bearing on the differential diagnosis. These themes are covered later in this chapter.

A comprehensive list of the potential infective causes of a fever is beyond the scope of this text. We will concentrate on broad themes and provide examples.

● Classification of fever

Common causes of fever presenting to emergency departments
- Viral infection – respiratory tract infection, influenza, infectious mononucleosis ('glandular fever' due to Epstein–Barr virus)
- Bacterial infection – commonly urinary tract infection, pneumonia, tonsillitis, cellulitis
- Parasitic infection – malaria in a traveller returned from an endemic area

Less common causes of fever
- Less common infections:
  - Bacterial (e.g. endocarditis, meningitis, cholangitis, pleural empyema, tuberculosis)
  - Viral (e.g. cytomegalovirus, hepatitis A)
  - Parasitic – usually in returned travellers (e.g. schistosomiasis)
  - Fungal – usually in immunosuppressed patients (e.g. aspergillosis)
- Multi-system inflammatory diseases:
  - Rheumatoid arthritis
  - Systemic lupus erythematosis (SLE)
  - Polymyalgia rheumatica/giant cell arteritis
  - Wegener's granulomatosis (ANCA-positive vasculitis)
- Malignancy:
  - Lymphoma
  - Leukaemia
  - Solid tumours (e.g. renal cell carcinoma)
- Sarcoidosis
- Drug-induced:
  - Rifampicin
  - Serotonin reuptake inhibitors (SSRIs)
  - Recreational drugs such as ecstasy – can be responsible for hyperthermia
- Inflammatory bowel disease

Rare causes of fever

- Familial Mediterranean fever
- Amyloidosis
- Adult Still's disease (see Chapter 17)
- Thyrotoxicosis
- Neuroleptic malignant syndrome

HAZARD

- Always consider the possibility of tuberculosis (TB) in patients with a fever of longer than two weeks' duration who were born in a high-incidence country, no matter how long they have been resident in a low-incidence country. This is because primary TB is usually contracted in childhood and may remain latent only to reactivate decades later. The most common cause of failure to diagnose TB is failure to consider the diagnosis as a possibility in the first place. *Late diagnosis in hospital can lead to exposure of other inpatients to potentially infectious cases of TB.*
- If you do suspect TB, then ask for urgent specialist advice from either a respiratory or an infectious diseases physician. High-incidence countries are those in Africa, the Indian subcontinent, South East Asia and some former Soviet countries such as Russia and Ukraine.

THINK

When does a fever become hyperthermia?
Technically, any fever can be defined as hyperthermia. The term is, however, usually reserved for core body temperatures exceeding 40.5°C. Although uncommon,

this is a medical emergency that carries a high mortality. Urgent action to cool the patient is required as multi-organ failure can result if the core temperature is elevated to this degree for a prolonged period. Causes include:

- heatstroke during excessively hot weather
- neuroleptic malignant syndrome
- ecstasy ingestion
- rarely, reactions to anaesthetic agents.

Those at increased risk of heatstroke include the elderly and patients with chronic medical conditions in whom thermoregulatory mechanisms may be impaired.

● History

First obtain a comprehensive history of the fever, paying careful attention to its duration and pattern, together with associated symptoms that may suggest a cause. Examples include dysuria due to urinary tract infection, cough due to pneumonia, and viral respiratory tract infection and sore throat due to pharyngitis.

CLINICAL TIP

In assessing a patient with a fever, *the context* is a vital part of the diagnostic reasoning process. Infection is the most likely cause and the context has a major bearing on the likely infective organisms.

- **Demographics** (age and location of the patient). The spectrum of infection will differ if the patient is a frail elderly nursing home resident (in whom urinary tract infections and pneumonia are common) compared with young healthy adults (in whom, for example, sexually transmitted infections must be considered).

- **Country of origin**. Always ask where a patient was born. If born in a country with a high incidence of TB, consider TB as a possible cause from the outset.
- **Immune status**. There are a number of different ways in which a patient can be immunosuppressed. The most immediately life-threatening scenario is neutropenic sepsis, of which the most common cause is cancer chemotherapy. Remember also that diabetic patients are at increased risk of infection. Consider whether the patient has identifiable loss of immune function from:
  - recent cancer chemotherapy
  - HIV infection
  - long-term corticosteroid therapy
  - chronic disease (e.g renal or liver failure)
  - diabetes
  - immunosuppressive drugs.
- **Lifestyle factors**. Some population groups have increased susceptibility to certain infections. Examples include lower gastrointestinal infections such as *Giardia* in men who have sex with men, and parenterally introduced staphylococcal infections in intravenous drug users. Always consider the possibility of HIV in these groups as well (see **Think** below). Take a history of recent unprotected sexual contacts unless this would be completely inappropriate.
- **Employment**. Some occupations involve exposure to organisms that are not seen commonly in the general population. Examples include brucellosis in farmers working with cattle, and leptospirosis in pest-control officers exposed to rats.
- **Hobbies**. Some recreational activities can lead to exposure to unusual organisms. Bird fanciers who keep parrots and other psittacine birds may be exposed to *Chlamydia psittaci*, which can cause psittacosis.

- **Travel**. A careful travel history is vital in any patient with a fever, for two reasons. First, potential causative organisms vary widely depending on the countries and areas visited. Second, some countries have a high incidence of microbial resistance to commonly used antibiotics. Examples include the high rate of amoxicillin resistance of *Streptococcus* species in Spain, and the extremely high rates of microbial resistance in India.
- **Drugs**. A full drug history is important, both of prescribed medications and recreational drug use. Intravenous drug abuse constitutes a major risk for infective endocarditis.

THINK

Who is at risk from HIV?
HIV is no longer confined to defined population groups as it was in the 1980s. Although some groups undoubtedly remain at increased risk, never make assumptions about an individual's risk (or lack of risk) of HIV infection. In addition, patients may not feel able to disclose behaviour that has put them at risk. An HIV test should be a routine part of the further investigation of unexplained fever and should be presented to the patient as such.

HAZARD

Fever in a neutropenic patient (defined as a neutrophil count $<0.5 \times 10^9/L$) is a medical emergency. Infection in this context can be rapidly overwhelming even when the patient appears stable at first presentation. Blood cultures should be taken and broad-spectrum intravenous antibiotics administered immediately according to your local neutropenic sepsis protocol.

● Examination

In a febrile patient the first concern is to establish whether any features of **severe sepsis** or **septic shock** are present. This topic is covered in more detail in Chapter 1.

- *Severe sepsis* can be defined as sepsis with sepsis-induced organ dysfunction. Mortality is 17–20 per cent.
- *Septic shock* can be defined as sepsis-induced hypotension persisting despite adequate fluid resuscitation. Mortality is 43–54 per cent.

Therefore, examine first for:

- blood pressure
- pulse rate
- respiratory rate
- peripheral perfusion (capillary refill time)
- oxygen saturation.

If the patient is haemodynamically unstable, fluid resuscitation and broad-spectrum intravenous antibiotics should be started immediately, with blood cultures drawn at the same time.

Look for a source of infection

- **Pharyngitis**. An inflamed pharynx or tonsils indicates possible streptococcal pharyngitis. Exudates or pus may be visible in the pharynx.
- **Sinusitis**. Facial pain and tenderness over the maxillary or frontal sinuses may indicate sinus infection.
- **Meningitis**. Examine for a stiff neck and photophobia (see Chapter 10 for a fuller description of these signs).
- **Pneumonia**. Auscultate the lungs for inspiratory crackles and bronchial breathing. Look also for evidence of a pleural effusion (dull percussion note and absent breath sounds). In the context of fever, this may indicate empyema formation, which requires prompt investigation and treatment.

- **Respiratory tract viral infection or bronchitis**. Auscultate the lungs for wheezing. Patients with underlying asthma or chronic obstructive pulmonary disease (COPD) will have a higher risk of developing a viral lower respiratory tract infection, but wheezing can occur in otherwise healthy subjects in this context as well.
- **Endocarditis**. Auscultate the heart for murmurs. The often-described peripheral manifestations of endocarditis (splinter haemorrhages, Roth spots in the fundi, Janeway lesions and Osler's nodes on the hands) should be looked for but they are rare in developed countries.
- **Intra-abdominal or pelvic sepsis**. Examine for abdominal tenderness and guarding. In pre-menopausal women, always consider the possibility of a retained tampon: *toxic-shock syndrome is a medical emergency*.
- **Renal tract infection**. Examine for loin and suprapubic tenderness.
- **Cellulitis**. Inspect the skin for tender red areas of cellulitis. If present, seek a local portal of entry for bacteria. Cellulitis of any area of the face is a particular emergency because of the risk of spread to adjacent vulnerable structures, particularly the eye and intracranial space (see **Hazard** below).

THINK

Where should one look for a portal of entry for bacteria in a case of cellulitis?
Most cases of cellulitis occur in the leg below the knee. Apart from an obvious injury causing a break in the skin or an insect bite, look for evidence of *Tinea pedis* between the toes. You will often find severe *Tinea* with cracked skin between the toes of patients with cellulitis. *Tinea* should be aggressively treated with oral and topical antifungal agents to help prevent a recurrence of cellulitis.

HAZARD

Facial cellulitis can spread to cause *orbital cellulitis*. This is a medical emergency that can lead to permanent eye damage with loss of sight. As well as prompt antibiotic treatment, a CT of the head is indicated to assess orbital involvement. Early specialist assessment by an ophthalmologist is also essential.

- **Abscesses**. Most patients will bring a painful fluctuant swelling to your attention without much prompting, but look carefully for a hot fluctuant swelling in a febrile patient who cannot communicate with you for any reason, for instance due to dysphasia or dementia.
- **Lymphadenopathy**. Check the cervical region, supraclavicular fossae, axillae and groins. Enlarged lymph nodes can indicate a variety of differential diagnoses, depending on their site, their size and whether or not they are painful. Possibilities are as follows.
  - *Reactive lymphadenopathy*. This is characterized by painful enlarged nodes in association with infection nearby.
  - *Viral infections*. Lymphadenopathy tends to be more generalized with viral infection. Infectious mononucleosis due to Epstein–Barr virus and HIV are examples.
  - *Tuberculosis*. Lymph node TB often involves the cervical lymph nodes and they are not usually hot or tender to touch. As stated above, consider the country of origin of the patient in your assessment of the likelihood of TB.
  - *Lymphoma*. Lymphadenopathy is usually painless and often described as 'rubbery'.
  - *Metastatic malignancy*. Involved lymph nodes are usually hard on palpation and commonly fixed to underlying tissue.

– *Sarcoidosis*. Pulmonary hilar nodes are those most commonly involved in sarcoidosis and they can be seen readily on chest x-ray. Peripheral lymphadenopathy is uncommon in sarcoidosis.

● **Uncommon sites of infection**. If no apparent source of infection can be identified, consider less common sources that are often overlooked. Examples include:
  – septic arthritis
  – osteomyelitis
  – 'discitis' of the spine
  – epidural abscess
  – pericardial infection.

● Investigations

The cause of a fever may be readily identifiable from the clinical history and examination findings. Often little or no further investigation will be indicated – an example is the patient presenting with a viral upper respiratory tract infection. However, in the secondary care setting, some investigations are usually indicated and most febrile patients presenting to emergency services will require the following.

● *Full blood count*. Look particularly at the White Cell and Neutrophil counts.
● *Blood cultures*.
● *Urea and electrolytes*.
● *Random blood glucose*. This is indicated in all patients whether they are known to be diabetic or not. Diabetes is frequently diagnosed in this setting.
● *Liver function tests*. These are often non-specifically deranged in acute sepsis but may also indicate acute hepatitis.
● *C-reactive protein*. Look for an acute phase response.
● *Urine dipstick for protein, blood and nitrites*. If present these abnormalities strongly support a diagnosis of urosepsis.

Microscopic haematuria can also be a feature of infective endocarditis.

- *Urine microscopy and culture.*
- *Chest radiography.* Look for evidence of pneumonia, pleural effusion or mediastinal lymphadenopathy.

Depending on the specific presentation of the patient, other initial investigations may be indicated as follows.

- *Stool microscopy and culture* – if the patient has diarrhoea.
- *Blood thick films* – for malaria in a returned traveller from a malaria endemic area. At least three films should be sent as the diagnosis is not always evident on the first sample.
- *Sputum microscopy and culture* – only if there is a productive cough. Remember to ask specifically for TB microscopy and culture if risk factors for TB are present.
- *Throat swab* – if exudates or pus are visible in the pharynx of a patient with a sore throat.
- *Pleural fluid aspiration* – if an effusion is present. It is important to exclude empyema. Fluid should be sent for microscopy and culture, including TB if risk factors are present. If the patient has pneumonia, test the pleural fluid pH: a pleural fluid pH below 7.2 is a reliable indicator of bacterial infection and the effusion should then be drained to dryness by means of a chest drain. If the pleural fluid is frankly purulent, a chest drain and respiratory specialist opinion is mandatory.
- *Lumbar puncture* – to obtain cerebrospinal fluid (CSF) for analysis if meningitis is suspected. A CT of the head may be indicated beforehand (see Chapter 10 for a full description of CSF analysis and indications for CT head scan).
- *Viral serology* – the spectrum of viruses tested for will depend on the clinical presentation. An exhaustive list of possibilities is beyond the scope of this text.
- *Serum creatine kinase* – if the patient is on neuroleptic drugs. A normal result rules out neuroleptic malignant syndrome.

- *Echocardiogram* – if infective endocarditis is suspected. A transthoracic echocardiogram is usually performed first. This may give suboptimal views of the valve leaflets, so a transoesophageal echocardiogram will be required if there is clinical suspicion of endocarditis. Several extra sets of blood cultures should be sent if endocarditis is suspected, preferably before antibiotics are administered.
- *Blood serum amylase/lipase levels*, depending on which is available in your laboratory – if abdominal pain or tenderness is present. Lipase levels rise in many causes of an 'acute abdomen' but are usually elevated at least five times above normal in pancreatitis.
- *Abdominal ultrasound or CT* – if intra-abdominal or pelvic sepsis is suspected. Ultrasound is usually sufficient to diagnose:
  - bile duct dilation
  - liver abscess
  - renal tract obstruction
  - renal abscess.

  CT is, however, superior in the diagnosis of:
  - pancreatitis
  - diverticular abscess
  - other intra-abdominal or pelvic sepsis.
- *Pelvic examination with high vaginal swab for microbiology* – indicated in females if sexually transmitted infection or other pelvic infection is suspected. The procedure should be carried out by either a gynaecologist or a genitourinary medicine physician.
- *Examination of the male genitalia* – with urethral and (if appropriate) rectal swabs for microbiology. This is the equivalent investigation in males if sexually transmitted infection is suspected. This should be carried out by a genitourinary medicine physician.

Further investigations in the case of a pyrexia of unknown origin

If the patient has not recovered despite empirical treatment and extensive investigation over the course of 2–3 weeks, then you are in 'PUO territory'. You may already have performed most of the investigations listed above. A detailed description of all possible causes of PUO and relevant investigations is beyond the scope of this text but, as a general guide, we would recommend considering the following.

- **Multi-system inflammatory diseases and vasculitis**. Send blood for a full autoantibody screen including ANA, ANCA, rheumatoid factor and anti-double-stranded DNA.
- **Tuberculosis**. Ask for specialist help from a respiratory physician or infectious disease specialist as to whether TB is a possibility and how it can be investigated. Do not place undue emphasis on the result of specific immune globulin tests for TB such as the QuantiFERON®-TB Gold test, as this is not a reliable way of 'ruling in' or 'ruling out' a diagnosis of active TB.
- **Malignancy**. Check whether you have adequately excluded tumours such as renal cell carcinoma, lymphoma and myeloma. In practice, this usually requires a CT scan of the chest, abdomen and pelvis, skeletal survey and blood tests for protein electrophoresis with urine for Bence Jones protein.
- **Other sources of sepsis**. Sources often overlooked by physicians are dental abscesses and sexually transmitted infections.
- **'Weird' infections**. Discuss the case with an infectious diseases specialist and check whether you have tested for anything rare that might be relevant given the patient's occupation, pets and hobbies.
- **Thyrotoxicosis**. Ensure that you have a recent set of thyroid function tests filed.

- **Factitious fever**. Some patients fabricate symptoms and, however unlikely this seems, the possibility will need to be considered on occasion. Suspicions may be raised if the patient is otherwise entirely well, has undergone a large number of normal investigations, and has a significant secondary gain to be obtained from being in hospital.

17 Joint problems

Introduction

The differential diagnosis of acutely painful joints can appear daunting, but application of a few basic principles will facilitate an effective clinical approach. In particular, it will ensure that potentially serious pathologies are investigated efficiently and quickly.

The predominating symptom may be *pain*, *stiffness*, *swelling* or *heat* – or any combination of these – and symptoms may be referrable to one or more joints. In the case of polyarthritis, the distribution of joint involvement provides useful information as to aetiology.

> ### ⚡ HAZARD
> Not all presentations with joint pain are due to joint pathology. Non-rheumatological conditions can mimic joint pain. Examples include hypertrophic pulmonary osteoarthropathy (HPOA), bone pain from secondary malignant deposits, a fracture adjacent to a joint, tendonitis, bursitis or soft tissue pain.

● Classification of acute arthropathy

Septic arthritis

- Approximately 70 per cent of cases in the UK are caused by staphylococcal infection.
- *Streptococcus* can also be responsible, and *Neisseria gonorrhoeae* is relatively common in the sexually active population.
- *Haemophilus* should be considered as the potential culprit in children.

Crystal arthritis

Joint aspiration is required in a search for crystals as follows:

- Birefringent uric acid crystals indicative of gout. Although serum uric acid is commonly elevated in acute gout, this is not invariably so and absence of birefringent crystals from joint fluid is necessary to exclude the diagnosis confidently.
- Pseudo-gout is characterized by the presence of calcium pyrophosphate crystals.
- Hydroxyapatite crystals are sometimes identified in elderly patients; the shoulder joints are commonly affected.

Traumatic arthritis

- The responsible trauma may be injury-related synovitis, anterior cruciate ligament rupture, or a fracture adjacent to (or possibly involving) a joint.
- Haemarthrosis is commonly secondary to trauma but can also arise spontaneously in the presence of a clotting disorder. Recurrent spontaneous haemarthrosis is a classical feature of haemophilia.

Reactive arthritis

- Reactive arthritis can be caused by a variety of infections, principally viruses and infectious diarrhoea. Potential causes include Coxsackie, Echo,

Epstein–Barr, rubella, hepatitis A and B, *Shigella*, *Salmonella* and *Campylobacter*. Knee and ankle joints are typically involved but a rheumatoid-type distribution is also seen.
- Parvovirus infection is another possibility in both children and adults.
- Reiter's syndrome is an uncommon type of reactive arthritis with a classical presentation.

Mono-articular presentations of inflammatory joint disease (examples)
- Rheumatoid arthritis
- Seronegative arthritides:
  - Psoriatic
  - Reactive (see above)
  - Ankylosing spondylitis
  - In association with inflammatory bowel disease
- Connective tissue disease:
  - Systemic lupus erythematosus (SLE)
  - Mixed connective tissue disease
  - Scleroderma
- Drugs: diuretics, antibiotics (quinolones) and cytotoxics can cause arthritis occasionally
- Rare causes:
  - Sarcoidosis
  - Rheumatic fever
  - Behçet's syndrome
  - Bacterial endocarditis
  - Henoch–Schönlein purpura
  - Familial Mediterranean fever
  - Adult Still's disease

Malignant tumours (rare)
- Synovioma, osteosarcoma
- Secondary deposit
- Hypertrophic pulmonary osteoarthropathy (HPOA)

THINK

What are the features of HPOA?
Carcinoma of the bronchus can rarely present with
acute periarticular pain due to hypertrophic pulmonary
osteoarthropathy, and this can mimic mono-arthritis or
polyarthritis. The symptoms are most common around
the knees, ankles and wrists, and there is a characteristic
appearance of subperiosteal calcification on x-ray.
Clubbing of the nails is invariably associated.

HAZARD

An acute mono-arthritis should be considered to be due
to sepsis until proved otherwise. The annual incidence of
septic arthritis is approximately 4 per 100 000 of the
population, and the consequences of missing this
diagnosis are serious. If sepsis is not treated promptly:

- approximately 50 per cent of cartilage is lost in 48 hours
- bone loss is evident in 7 days
- a significant mortality accrues – this has been quoted
  at 10–15 per cent overall.

CLINICAL TIP

The most important investigations if septic arthritis is
suspected are:

- pre-antibiotic blood cultures
- culture of synovial fluid from the offending joint when
  at all possible.

History

Septic arthritis

- Enquire about risk factors, including systemic reasons for
  immunosuppression (e.g. malignant disease, chemotherapy

or HIV infection) and diabetes. In addition, local joint pathology can predispose to infection. Rheumatoid arthritis is the classic example, but degenerative joints are also more prone to becoming infected.

- Septic arthritis is particularly likely at extremes of age but, in sexually active individuals, ask for any symptoms of sexually transmitted infections.
- A joint prosthesis is always potentially vulnerable to organisms introduced into the circulation during invasive medical procedures. Enquire about recent invasive procedures (cystoscopy, colonoscopy especially) in anyone who has pain and/or swelling related to a prosthetic joint.

Crystal arthritis

- Previous episodes of arthritis are common, so ask whether the current episode is the first, or whether there has been a recurrent history.
- Ask for risk factors for gout, including:
  - excess alcohol
  - a high-protein (high purine content) diet
  - drugs, especially diuretics
  - high cell-turnover states (e.g. lymphoproliferative disorders and psoriasis).
- The pyrophosphate crystals of pseudo-gout are shed from damaged cartilage and osteoarthritis is a common precursor. It occurs more commonly in women and the knee is the joint most commonly affected.
- Hydroxyapatite crystal arthropathy is more common in the elderly, and the synovial shedding of these crystals is recognized in 'renal dialysis' arthropathy.

Traumatic arthritis

Ask carefully about any episodes of trauma, but remember the possibility of stress fractures (with no history of trauma) in the elderly and malnourished.

Reactive arthritis

- Enquire about a preceding illness suggestive of viral infection or infectious diarrhoea, which may have occurred up to three weeks previously.
- Reiter's syndrome is a reactive arthropathy with a classical presentation (see **Clinical tip** below).
- Enquire also about a preceding history of diarrhoea. *Shigella*, *Salmonella*, *Campylobacter* and *Yersinia* gastrointestinal infections are all recognized to be precursors of reactive arthritis.

Interestingly, affected individuals are often HLA B27-positive and, if so, they are more likely to develop recurrent arthropathy and may even progress to chronic arthritis.

CLINICAL TIP

The classical combination of clinical features in *Reiter's syndrome* is:

- seronegative asymmetric arthritis that commonly involves the lower limbs, though swelling of proximal interphalangeal joints can occur
- urethritis or cervicitis
- the characteristic skin rash of keratoderma blenorrhagica

However, it is quite common for the syndrome not to manifest all of these features. Sexual transmission is associated and certain social events may be related – an example was an outbreak associated with young adult holidays to Ibiza.

Inflammatory joint disease

Recurrent symptoms will raise suspicion and a careful history of any preceding episodes is important.

- Rheumatoid arthritis affects women three times more than men. The distribution of joint involvement classically includes the small joints of the hands and feet, commonly with a degree of joint deformity. However, remember that other connective tissue diseases are more common in women and may manifest in identical joint involvement.

- It is important to enquire for evidence of *systemic* disease, including:
    - skin rashes, upper GI symptoms and skin manifestations of scleroderma
    - episodes of pleuritic chest pain in association with systemic lupus erythematosis (SLE).
- The joint distribution of seronegative arthritis tends to be different with large joint pathology, involvement of interphalangeal joints and sacroiliitis being classical.
- Look for a skin rash suggestive of psoriasis.
- Enquire about symptoms suggestive of inflammatory bowel disease. These are commonly present at the same time as joint symptoms, although arthropathy can precede active bowel inflammation.
- The classical natural history of ankylosing spondylitis involves lower back pain and early morning stiffness. Peripheral joint involvement occurs in approximately 40 per cent of individuals and uveitis is occasionally associated. Young adult males are typically affected.

● Examination

Your examination can be structured in an identical way to the history in order to narrow the differential diagnosis.

Septic arthritis
- Any joint can be involved and a mono-arthritis is the most common presentation, although multiple joints may become infected (e.g. in staphylococcal septicaemia and with gonococcal disease).
- Affected joints will be hot, swollen and often red.
- Pressing on the joint line commonly causes pain.
- Look for systemic signs of sepsis such as fever, tachycardia and hypotension.

Crystal arthritis

- Gout can affect many joints, but ankles, wrists, elbows and first metatarsal joints are classically involved. Look for extra-articular deposits of uric acid (tophi). These may be periarticular or seen in the pinnae of the ear or adjacent to nasal cartilage.
- Pseudo-gout usually affects large joints, most commonly the knee.

Traumatic arthritis

Examine for additional signs of trauma.

Reactive arthritis

- Look for skin rashes. A number of viruses can cause a rash in association with acute joint pain. Examples include parvovirus and rubella, although the rash of parvovirus may precede the joint symptoms by 2–3 weeks.
- Look for evidence of infection with other viruses – Epstein–Barr virus (lymphadenopathy), hepatitis A and B (jaundice).

Viral reactive arthritis most commonly affects the knees and ankles.

- There may be evidence of bowel pathology when arthritis is associated with *Salmonella*, *Yersinia*, *Shigella* or *Campylobacter* infections; but, again, gut symptoms and signs may antedate joint pathology and no longer be present when joint symptoms arise.
- In particular, look for evidence of sexually transmitted disease with oral and/or genital ulceration and specifically for eye involvement (conjunctivitis and iritis) and the characteristic skin rash (keratoderma blenorrhagica) of Reiter's syndrome.

Inflammatory joint disease

Rheumatoid arthritis

All synovial joints can be involved in rheumatoid arthritis and, although the typical manifestation is a symmetrical polyarthritis affecting the small joints of the hands and feet, rheumatoid arthritis can present as a relapsing or persistent mono-arthritis.

Look for extra-articular manifestations of rheumatoid disease, including subcutaneous nodules, lymphadenopathy, anaemia, episcleritis, pulmonary fibrosis, pleural effusion(s) and pericarditis.

Other connective tissue diseases
Look for multi-system signs suggestive of SLE, including skin rashes and pleurisy. Look also for the typical facial and hand changes of scleroderma.

CLINICAL TIP

Extra-articular manifestations in connective tissue disease include the following.

- *Pleuritic chest pain* is common in SLE. Characteristically, pleuritic chest pain is prominent, but pleural effusions – if present – are generally small. This is in contrast to rheumatoid pleural disease where pain is usually not marked and the effusions can be very large.
- In *scleroderma*, the characteristic skin changes of the hand are summarized as: C (calcinosis of the fingers), R (Raynaud's phenomenon), S (sclerodactyly) and T (telangiectasia). When combined with the oesophageal manifestations of scleroderma, this becomes the 'CREST' syndrome.

Psoriatic arthropathy
- The distribution of joint involvement is very variable, from a mono- or asymmetrical oligo-arthritis to a symmetrical polyarthritis, which may resemble rheumatoid arthritis.
- Look carefully for the tell-tale skin rash, classically on the extensor aspects of the limbs; but remember also to look in unusual sites – the scalp, behind the ears and in the umbilicus.

- Nail changes also offer a clue as to diagnosis, and nail 'pitting' is very common. The more dramatic changes of onycholysis are also occasionally seen.

Inflammatory bowel disease
- Look for the perianal manifestations of Crohn's disease, including anal tags and fistulae as well as mouth ulcers.
- Erythema nodosum is occasionally seen in association and iritis may also accompany this syndrome of 'enteropathic' arthritis.

Miscellaneous diagnoses
The following conditions can all be associated with joint disease.

Bacterial endocarditis
Listen for murmurs. Look for extra-cardiac manifestations of endocarditis, including:

- splinter haemorrhages in the nails
- Osler's nodes and Janeway lesions in the hands (both rare)
- Roth spots on fundoscopy (rare)
- splenomegaly
- haematuria.

Rheumatic fever
Now very uncommon in industrialized societies, this post-streptococcal condition characteristically causes an arthritis that:

- 'flits' from one joint to another
- may be associated with the classical (though rare) skin rash of erythema marginatum
- is associated with heart murmurs.

Henoch–Schönlein purpura
Arthritis can occur in association with the classical purpuric skin rash affecting the legs and buttocks. Other manifestations are:

- haematuria
- abdominal pain
- intestinal bleeding (rarely).

Sarcoidosis

Most common in – but far from exclusive to – young adults, sarcoidosis usually affects the ankle joints, although wrists and knees are other common sites of joint pathology. Erythema nodosum is classically associated, and the full combination includes bilateral hilar lymphadenopathy on chest x-ray, when there can be little doubt about the diagnosis.

Familial Mediterranean fever

This unusual condition is a hereditary inflammatory disorder that affects groups of people originating from around the Mediterranean Sea. It is prominently present in the Armenian people, Sephardic Jews and, to a lesser extent, in Ashkenazi Jews, Greeks, and people from Turkey and the Arab countries. The arthritis is usually mono-articular and the recurrent episodes are also characterized by fever, abdominal pain and, sometimes, pleurisy.

Behçet's syndrome

Interestingly, the geographical distribution of this rare condition is similar to that of Familial Mediterranean Fever. Painful oral and genital ulceration is the clue to the diagnosis. There are a number of eye conditions that may occur, with iritis being the most common.

Adult Still's disease

This is a fascinating and rare condition offering a challenging diagnosis. The cervical spine, wrists and large joints of the lower limbs are typically involved. Accompanying features on history and examination are:

- an evanescent, salmon-pink skin rash associated with spikes of fever, which are common in the evening
- episodes of pericarditis and pleuritic chest pain
- lymphadenopathy and splenomegaly (may not be present).

Investigations are important in supporting the clinical diagnosis. A neutrophil leucocytosis is the norm, serum ferritin is commonly elevated and transaminases may be elevated too. Blood cultures and rheumatoid factor are negative.

● Investigations

Synovial fluid aspiration

The indications for joint aspiration are:

- potential septic arthritis
- potential crystal arthritis
- potential haemarthrosis
- relief of symptoms.

In practice, the default position will be to aspirate a swollen joint unless there is a contraindication, although in some circumstances a request for specialist help with the procedure will be appropriate. Synovial fluid should be sent for:

- white cell count
- microbiology
- polarized microscopy, looking for crystals.

Blood tests

- *Full blood count*:
  - Haemoglobin may be low in chronic diseases (e.g. rheumatoid arthritis).
  - White cell count is elevated in many causes of arthropathy (septic, inflammatory and reactive), but a very high white cell count ($>18\,000/mm^3$) should raise suspicion of infection.
- *Inflammatory markers:*
  - Both C-reactive protein (CRP) and ESR are typically elevated in septic arthritis but are raised in various forms of inflammatory joint disease as well.
  - In SLE, it is quite common to see a normal CRP in the presence of a high ESR and this discrepant finding may aid diagnosis.
  - An elevated serum ferritin is typically seen in Adult Still's disease.
- *Renal and liver function tests*. These should be checked routinely. Abnormalities may be seen in general systems

disorders (e.g. SLE) but may also be an indicator of multi-organ problems in sepsis.

- *Blood cultures.* These are mandatory.
- *Blood glucose and uric acid.* These should be checked to look for diabetes and gout.
- *Blood clotting screen.* Any abnormality may indicate a bleeding diathesis and predisposition to haemarthrosis, and should prompt a haematological referral.
- *Immunological investigations:*
  - Rheumatoid factor and antinuclear antibodies should be requested. If positive they suggest inflammatory arthritis, but they are not specific for individual connective tissue diseases.
  - Positive anti-double-stranded DNA antibodies, however, are highly specific for SLE.
  - Extractable nuclear antigen consists of a mix of nuclear antigens, and the details of relevant positivity can help to narrow the diagnosis in connective tissue diseases (Table 17.1).

Table 17.1 Relevance of individual antibody tests in connective tissue disease

Antibody	Association
Rheumatoid factor	<ul><li>Rheumatoid arthritis</li><li>40% cases of SLE</li><li>Non-specific elevation in a number of inflammatory disorders</li></ul>
Antinuclear antibody	SLE and other autoimmune disorders
Anti-ds-DNA	SLE
ENA	
• Anti-RNP	• Mixed connective tissue disease, SLE
• Ro	• Primary Sjogren's, SLE
• La	• Primary Sjogren's
• Anti-smooth muscle	• SLE, chronic active hepatitis
• Anti-centromere	• Limited systemic sclerosis
• SCL-70	• Diffuse systemic sclerosis
• Jo-1	• Polymyositis
• Anti-cardiolipin	• SLE, anti-phospholipid syndrome

SLE, systemic lupus erythematosis; ds-DNA, double-stranded deoxyribonucleic acid; ENA, extractable nuclear antigen; RNP, ribonucleoprotein

- *HLA testing.* HLA B27 genotype is common in individuals with ankylosing spondylitis and in enteropathic arthritis. It is also interesting that HLA B27 positivity is more common in those with reactive arthritis following infection with a number of micro-organisms, including *Chlamydia*, *Shigella*, *Salmonella*, *Campylobacter* and *Yersinia*. Moreover, the possession of this genotype seems to make progression to a more chronic arthropathy after a reactive event more likely.

Sepsis screen

This should include a chest x-ray and mid-stream urine. Skin pustules (e.g. in gonococcal septicaemia) should be aspirated and cultured. Urethral and cervical swabs should be taken if appropriate.

Further investigations

- *X-rays* should be taken of affected joints. Chondrocalcinosis is typical of pseudo-gout, and characteristic changes of rheumatoid arthritis (cysts and/or periarticular osteoporosis) are diagnostic.
- Periarticular fractures are sometimes invisible on x-ray, so *isotope bone scanning* may be indicated.

HAZARD

In *septic arthritis* there may be no radiographic abnormalities for up to two weeks. Normal x-ray studies do not exclude this diagnosis, so we emphasize the early statement of this chapter: *an acute mono-arthritis should be considered to be due to sepsis until proved otherwise.* The priority and promptness of your investigations should reflect this imperative.

18 Skin rashes

● Introduction

This chapter cannot provide an exhaustive account of dermatological differential diagnosis. Rather, it is designed to provide a systematic approach to the patient presenting to emergency services with a skin rash. Rash may be the sole reason for the patient's presentation or it may be just one of the manifestations of a non-dermatological clinical problem. The emphasis throughout this chapter is on recognition of clinical conditions that are worrying and therefore the priority is to identify particular features of a rash that might indicate severe disease.

Note on the following classification of rashes

Our classification is geared to the 'front door' and is intended to assist you in structuring your clinical history and examination.

- First, do the appearances suggest a primarily epidermal process or a dermal one?
- Second, consider the differential diagnosis of blisters and pustules.
- Third, question the possibility of bacterial, viral or fungal infection.
- Finally, consider the possibility of insect bites or infestations.

● Classification of rashes in the acute medical setting

Epidermal origin

- Psoriasis
- Eczema
- Lichen planus
- Seborrhoeic dermatitis
- Pityriasis rosea
- Erythroderma
- Lupus erythematosus
- Keratoderma blenorrhagica (associated with reactive arthritis)

Dermal origin

- The erythemas
  - Erythema multiforme
  - Erythema nodosum
  - Erythema induratum
  - Drug reactions – generalized or 'fixed'
- Vasculitis (petechiae and purpura)
  - Meningococcal infection
  - Streptococcal infection
  - Henoch–Schönlein purpura
  - Drug reactions
  - Connective tissue diseases
  - Lymphoma and leukaemia
  - Dysproteinaemias
- Urticaria
  - Allergic
  - Angio-oedema
  - Physical – dermatographism, pressure, heat, cold, cholinergic, aquagenic

Blisters and pustules

- Widespread:
  - Chickenpox (Varicella)
  - Erythema multiforme

- Drug eruptions
- Generalized eczema
- Pemphigoid
- Pemphigus
- Dermatitis herpetiformis
- Localized:
  - Herpes zoster ('shingles')
  - Herpes simplex
  - Allergic reaction – insect bite, topical medication
  - Impetigo
  - Eczema – pompholyx

Bacterial infections

- Cellulitis, including erysipelas
- Pustules as a result of septicaemia
- Generalized rash in response to a local infection and with systemic toxin production (e.g. scarlet fever and toxic shock syndrome)
- Uncommon – tuberculosis, leprosy, opportunist mycobacteria

Viral infections

- Herpes simplex
- Herpes zoster
- Molluscum contagiosum – usually in infants but may be florid in immunocompromised adults
- Measles
- Rubella
- Hand, foot and mouth disease (Coxsackie A)

HIV infection

- Transient maculo–papular erythema as part of the conversion syndrome
- Herpes zoster – can be florid, with systemic spread
- Fungal infection
- Psoriasis is more common in HIV patients

- Mycobacterial infection
- Kaposi's sarcoma

Fungal infections

Nutritional disorders

Examples are pellagra (nicotinic acid deficiency) and scurvy (vitamin C deficiency). These conditions are rare in developed countries but are occasionally seen in elderly patients or people following extremely restricted diets.

Bites and infestations

This is a restricted list to reflect the likely exposure in the UK to indigenous problems and those related to returning travellers.

- Scabies (always consider this diagnosis in patients with excoriated skin from scratching. It is well-documented in patients from residential institutions and rough sleepers and is highly contagious.)
- Typhus
- Cutaneous leishmaniasis
- Lyme disease
- Dengue fever
- Spider bites

Dermatological terminology

- *Macule* – a change in skin colour with no elevation above the surrounding skin. The change may reflect increased melanin (blue or black colouration) or reduced melanin (white patches), or it may be pink or red owing to the subcutaneous vascular dilatation of inflammation.
- *Papules and nodules* – circumscribed, raised lesions. Papules are, by definition, less than 1 cm in diameter and nodules greater than 1 cm.

- *Vesicles and bullae* – raised lesions that contain fluid. They may be limited to the epidermis (e.g. pemphigus and epidermolysis bullosa), when they readily slough, or be dermal in site (pemphigoid).
- *Wheal* – a rounded raised lesion that is transient, disappearing within 24–48 hours. It is caused by oedema in the dermis. A rash consisting of wheals is *urticaria*.
- *Pustules* – vesicles containing purulent material, which may be infected (staphylococcal and gonococcal sepsis) or sterile as in pustular psoriasis.
- *Discoid* (or 'nummular') *lesions* – coin-like lesions of variable size, well defined and not very raised. They are usually an eczematous reaction.
- *Plaques* – slightly raised, often relatively large with well-defined edges. They tend to be 'figured' (likened to the inscription on a commemorative plaque) and have a propensity for scaling. This is typical of epidermal pathology and the classic example is psoriasis.
- *Lichenification* – the term comes from the natural appearance of lichen on rocks and trees. Skin is thickened and hardened with accentuated markings. This is usually a feature of prolonged skin rubbing in localized areas of eczema.
- *Annular lesions* – ring-shaped lesions that have clearer centres and may or may not have raised peripheries. Erythema multiforme and psoriasis are examples.

Potentially serious disease

Sometimes, the characteristics of the rash suggest either serious associated medical problems or a rash that has serious consequences in its own right. Alarm bells should ring with the following morphological features, and with particular anatomical and physiological observations.

Morphological features

- **Sepsis**. This may be:
  - indicative of a specific infection, such as meningococcal (non-blanching petechial rash first seen in pressure

areas), gonococcal (pustular lesions on the limbs perhaps with joint pain and swelling) or staphylococcal (may be similar pustular lesions)
- a generalized erythema of bacterial infection with systemic toxin release, such as scarlet fever secondary to a streptococcal sore throat, and the striking erythema of the 'toxic-shock' syndrome, one of the causes of which is a retained tampon in a woman of menstruating age
- a generalized rash with vesicles, such as disseminated herpes simplex or varicella zoster and drug eruptions (see **Hazard** below)
- infection in a traveller, such as the maculopapular rash of Dengue fever
- infection in association with immunocompromised states, such as Kaposi's sarcoma in AIDS, associated with human herpes virus subtype 8.

- **Anaphylaxis**. This is typically an urticarial rash in the presence of systemic features of anaphylaxis.
- **Systemic disease**. Examples are connective tissue diseases and vasculitides.
- **Potentially exfoliating skin diseases**. These are either primary or secondary skin problems that are characterized by extensive skin involvement with exfoliation. This is effectively 'acute skin failure' and is a medical emergency. The alerting features can be classified as follows:
  - generalized red rash with scaling: exfoliative erythroderma (may be a reaction to drugs)
  - generalized red rash with pustules: pustular psoriasis and drug eruptions
  - generalized red rash with blisters (often with prominent mouth lesions): erythema multiforme, toxic epidermal necrolysis, pemphigus, bullous pemphigoid and drug eruptions
- **Generalized purpura**. Consider:
  - thrombocytopaenia
  - disseminated intravascular coagulation, associated with a wide range of serious disease: sepsis, obstetric

complications, disseminated malignancy and major trauma

- vasculitis, including Henoch–Schönlein purpura
- meningococcaemia
- gonococcaemia
- bacterial endocarditis
- drug eruptions.

Physiological and anatomical considerations

- **Fever** – implies infection.
- **Systemic haemodynamic disturbance** – implies an associated shock state.
- **Exfoliation risk** – extensive Stevens–Johnson syndrome, or extensive bullous rashes such as pemphigus.
- **Anatomical distributions of the rash** – ophthalmic herpes zoster and bacterial facial cellulitis with its propensity to spread involving orbital and even intracranial structures.

HAZARD

Severe Varicella can occasionally be complicated by pneumonitis in adults which can be life-threatening. In this circumstance the extent of the vesicular skin rash is matched by the severity of the accompanying viral pneumonitis. This is an important alerting feature to the risk of respiratory failure and the need for supportive ventilation.

CLINICAL TIP

Generalized purpura that is palpable is a worrying clinical sign. It is usually due to vasculitis (including bacterial endocarditis) or meningococcaemia.

● History

Be systematic with your history:

Exogenous or endogenous aetiology?
Look for evidence of:

- an exogenous cause for the rash (e.g. infection)
- an endogenous condition (e.g. psoriasis or eczema).

What is the age of onset?
- Eczema tends to start in early life.
- Psoriasis begins usually in early adult life but can occur at any time from infancy to old age.
- Bullous pemphigoid affects older people.
- Pemphigus is a condition of middle age.

Have there been previous skin problems?
- If so, then an endogenous cause is more likely.
- If not, consider infection, infestation, contact dermatitis or another exogenous cause. There are exceptions: psoriasis can appear in older adults with no previous history.

Is there a history of other medical illness?
Examples are:

- atopic asthma in association with eczema
- coeliac disease with dermatitis herpetiformis
- connective tissue disease with vasculitic skin lesions
- various rashes associated with thyroid disease – pretibial myxoedema (hyperthyroidism) or the coarse dry skin of hypothyroidism.

Are others affected?
Are other individuals affected, at home, at school or at work? If so, consider a contagious condition such as scabies.

What is the distribution of the rash?
- What was the distribution at onset?
- How did it subsequently develop and spread?

Is there a history of contact with potentially sensitizing topical agents?

Examples are:

- contact dermatitis of the dominant hand in hairdressers, caused by scissors
- dermatitis of both hands in healthcare workers, caused by latex gloves
- facial dermatitis, following the use of new cosmetics or soap
- rash on the neck, associated with jewellery.

Take a medications history

This should include prescribed and over-the-counter medications, including homeopathic remedies.

Are there associated symptoms?

- Itching is common with the urticarias, eczema and lichen planus.
- Fever will suggest infection.
- Headache, myalgia and general symptoms point to viral or other infections.

Is there a family history of skin disease?

- If one parent has psoriasis, children have approximately a 25 per cent chance of developing the condition. If both parents are affected, this figure rises to 50 per cent, suggesting an autosomal dominant gene with partial penetrance.
- There is often also a positive family history in eczema.

Has there been a precipitating life event?

- Psoriasis can be precipitated by stress, including infection and childbirth.
- Eczema can be exacerbated by stressful events.

Is there anything to suggest a nutritional or vitamin deficiency?

Examples are scurvy and pellagra.

● Examination

Symmetry

- Most endogenous rashes affect both sides of the body, while exogenous rashes may be symmetrical or asymmetrical.
- Infections can be either localized or widespread.
- Contact dermatitis may show a distribution that reflects the area of contact: examples are given above in History.

Distribution

Be aware of the typical distribution of common skin conditions and common infections (Table 18.1). Figs 18.1–18.6 show typical distributions.

- Is the rash predominant in exposed areas of skin? If so, consider a relationship to sunlight (see **Think** below).
- Look for involvement in particular sites:
  - the classical skin burrows in the web spaces between the fingers in scabies
  - the scalp in psoriasis

Table 18.1 Characteristics of common viral exanthems

German measles (Rubella)	Pink macules on the face spreading to the trunk and limbs over 24–48 h
Measles (Variola)	One of the earliest signs in a pyrexial, 'grizzling' child is Koplik's spots (white spots surrounded by erythema) on the oral mucosa
	After about 48 h, a macular rash develops on the face, trunk and limbs
	Look for early lesions behind the ears
Chickenpox (Varicella)	Widespread 'cropping' of skin lesions over several days: lesions coexist at different stages of evolution from erythematous papules to vesicles to pustules to crusting
	The rash is widespread affecting the trunk, face, scalp, limbs and external genitalia
	Lesions are itchy, and scratching can result in unpleasant scarring

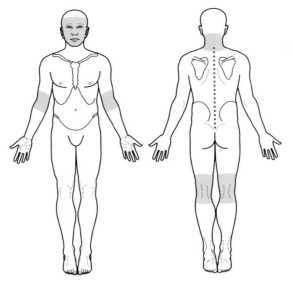

Fig. 18.1 Distribution of atopic eczema

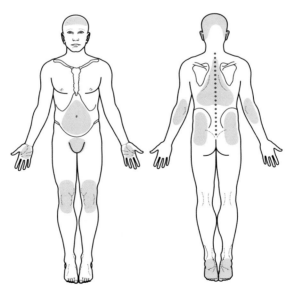

Fig. 18.2 Distribution of psoriasis

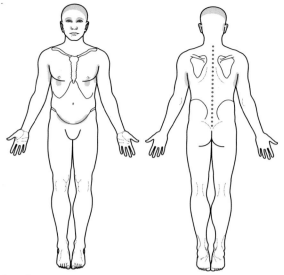

Fig. 18.3 Distribution of seborrhoeic dermatitis

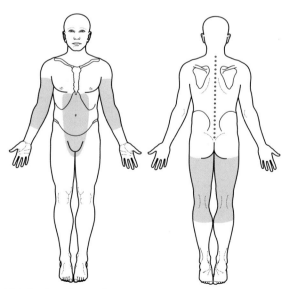

Fig. 18.4 Distribution of pemphigus

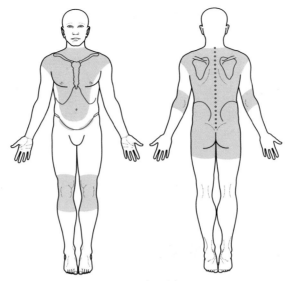

Fig. 18.5 Distribution of bullous pemphigoid

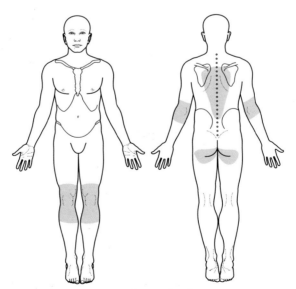

Fig. 18.6 Distribution of dermatitis herpetiformis

- palms and soles in psoriasis (when the lesions are often pustular)
- palms and soles in keratoderma blenorrhagica (associated with genital lesions and reactive arthritis) and also in secondary syphilis (maculo-papular)
- anterior shins in erythema nodosum and pretibial myxoedema (a rare association of hyperthyroidism)
- at sites of minor trauma, including scars, in psoriasis (Koebner's phenomenon)
- pressure areas (may be the first site of appearance of the non-blanching petechial skin rash of meningococcal septicaemia).

THINK

Why may a rash be related to sunlight?
A rash may be due to:
- sunlight alone (e.g. polymorphous light eruption)
- photosensitivity to topically applied substances
- photosensitivity to drugs taken internally.
Psoriatic lesions are often improved by sun exposure.

Morphology

Are the appearances more suggestive of epidermal or of dermal pathology?
Epidermal diseases are characterized by:

- thickening of the keratin layer and scaling – psoriasis
- lichenification, which is a more extensive and uniform area of thickening caused by rubbing – eczema
- small epidermal vesicles with crusting – eczema

Dermal lesions may be covered by normal epidermis. This is characteristic of many types of erythema where there is dilatation and inflammation of dermal blood vessels.

What is the nature of the rash margins?

- Well-defined margins are seen in psoriatic plaques.
- In eczema, the margins tend to merge into normal skin.

Are there vesicles and/or blisters?

- The vesicles of eczema and contact dermatitis are caused by oedema between epidermal cells, but this appearance may be overshadowed by inflammation and scaling.
- The large blisters (bullae) of pemphigus are caused by antibodies to the epidermis above the basement membrane. As a result there is separation of the epidermal cells and the superficial blister is very prone to separate. Even rubbing apparently normal skin can result in separation of the epidermis (Nikolsky's sign). Mucous membranes are commonly involved in pemphigus and are a clue to the diagnosis.

> ### THINK
>
> *What is the differential diagnosis of mouth ulceration in association with a skin rash?*
> Herpes simplex; erythema multiforme; trauma (e.g. dentures); pemphigus; lichen planus; hand, foot and mouth disease.

- The antibodies responsible for pemphigoid are directed at the upper layer of the basement membrane at the dermo-epidermal junction and, as a result, the blisters that form are deeper, tenser and less likely to burst. The distribution of the rash is different from pemphigus (see Figs 18.4 and 18.5) and mucosal involvement is not a feature.
- The blisters associated with bacterial infection (impetigo and specific septicaemias) tend to be more localized, as do the vesicles and blisters of herpes simplex (oral and genital involvement with types I and II, respectively) and shingles (dermatomal distribution). The distribution of the blisters

of chickenpox and of hand, foot and mouth disease are also helpful in diagnosis (see Table 18.1 on p. 261).

- In dermatitis herpetiformis, the blisters have a characteristic distribution over the knees, elbows, buttocks and back (see Fig. 18.6).

Is there induration and thickening of the skin?
This may be caused by:

- cell infiltration – mycosis fungoides, malignant secondary deposits
- granuloma formation – sarcoid, tuberculosis and other mycobacterial infections
- deposits of fat or amyloid.

Are there specific morphological appearances?
Specific morphological appearances that can help to make the diagnosis are:

- 'target' lesions of erythema multiforme
- teardrop lesions of 'guttate' psoriasis
- the characteristic migrating margins of erythema chronicum migrans (Lyme disease).

Purpura is defined as 'a circumscribed deposit of blood >5 mm in diameter' (petechiae are <5 mm). Purpura has a differential diagnosis of its own.

THINK

What is the differential diagnosis of purpura?
Thrombocytopenia; meningococcal septicaemia; gonococcal septicaemia; leukocytoclastic vasculitis, including Henoch–Schönlein purpura; rickettsial diseases, especially Rocky Mountain spotted fever; senile traumatic purpura.

Additional, specific organ involvement

Look for:

- nail pitting and arthropathy in psoriasis
- arthritis and genital lesions in keratoderma blenorrhagica
- arthropathy, pleural and pericardial disease in association with the vasculitic skin lesions (look in the nail beds) of systemic lupus erythematosis (SLE)
- appearances of sclerodactyly, telangiectasia and calcinosis in the digits and oesophageal pathology in scleroderma
- eye and joint involvement in erythema nodosum associated with sarcoidosis.

● Investigations

Blood tests

- *Full blood count.* Look for anaemia, white cell count abnormalities suggestive of infection and note the platelet count; especially in thrombocytopenic purpura.
- *Clotting screen.* This is useful as a general screen for clotting abnormalities and to look for disseminated intravascular coagulation (DIC).
- *C-reactive protein.* Use CRP as a marker of an inflammatory disease.
- *Erythrocyte sedimentation rate.* The ESR is elevated in connective tissue diseases when CRP may be normal.
- *Renal and liver function tests.* Use as general screening investigations.
- *Blood cultures* (a routine requirement).
- *Culture of other sites as appropriate.* Examples are CSF, joint fluid and aspiration of skin pustules. Scrapings of the petechial lesions of meningococcaemia smeared on a slide are a sensitive way to detect the organism after Gram staining.
- *Other blood tests.* These will depend on the presentation:
  - auto-immune profile
  - blood sugar

- thyroid function tests
- vasculitis screen
- specific viral and rickettsial antibodies.

Chest x-ray

Look for changes compatible with sarcoidosis, tuberculosis and connective tissue disease.

Urinalysis

Look for evidence of infection, and for microscopy changes (haematuria and casts) suggestive of vasculitic renal involvement.

Skin biopsy

May be required for a definitive diagnosis.

Dermatological opinion

Finally, in cases of diagnostic uncertainty or where you suspect significant primary skin disease, seek an early dermatological opinion.

19 Back pain

● Introduction

Back pain is an extremely common presenting complaint in acute medicine. Most episodes consist of lower back pain which is acute and self-limiting, often related to minor trauma such as heavy lifting. To put this in perspective, 84 per cent of adults will experience an episode of acute low back pain of this type at some point in their life. Although not considered medically 'sinister' or 'serious', such episodes can be temporarily disabling and distressing for patients. The diagnostic art lies in differentiating the minority of cases with a significant or serious underlying diagnosis, which is not self-limiting, from the majority who do not require specific investigation.

● History

The history is crucial in differentiating the minority of cases with a serious underlying diagnosis from the majority with self-limiting mechanical back pain. Enquire about the following.

- **Site**. Most back pain (and nearly all self-limiting back pain) is situated in the lower back. Thoracic or cervical spine pain is more likely to indicate a serious cause.
- **Onset**. Duration of pain and rapidity of onset are important features in differential diagnosis.
  - Sudden onset suggests disc prolapse, a vascular event (e.g. aortic dissection or an expanding or leaking

● Classification of back pain

Mechanical causes

- Trauma (includes heavy lifting)
- Poor posture and seating
- Spondylolisthesis
- Spondylosis
- Facet joint arthritis
- Spinal stenosis
- Lumbar disc prolapse – often following bending or lifting, and most commonly of L4/L5 and L5/S1 discs

Serious or sinister causes

- Malignancy:
  - Bony metastases
  - Myeloma
  - Primary bone tumours (rare)
- Metabolic:
  - Osteoporosis with vertebral crush fracture
- Inflammatory causes:
  - Rheumatoid arthritis
  - Seronegative arthritides (e.g. ankylosing spondylitis, psoriatic arthritis)
- Infection:
  - Osteomyelitis/discitis, including tuberculosis
  - Epidural abscess
- Referred from retroperitoneal structures:
  - Acute pyelonephritis
  - Renal stone
  - Pancreatitis
  - Abdominal aortic aneurysm
  - Aortic dissection

abdominal aortic aneurysm), or a fracture including those related to osteoporosis.

– Pain evolving over days or weeks is typical of malignancy.
– Inflammatory back pain usually presents with a longer history of weeks' or months' duration.
– Many patients with simple mechanical back pain have a history of recurrent episodes and a relevant recent episode of activity such as heavy lifting.
– Alternatively, there may be a relevant occupational history.

- **Radiation**. Nerve root entrapment (often referred to as radiculopathy or 'sciatica') can be caused by lateral disc prolapse in the lumbar spine. There is commonly a history of bending or lifting followed by sudden onset of back pain and muscle spasm associated with shooting pains and paraesthesiae and/or numbness radiating down one leg. There may be associated loss of tendon reflexes.

- **Bladder/bowel function**. Sphincter dysfunction (that is to say, urinary retention and/or constipation) occurring in the context of back pain is of vital significance and should prompt urgent investigation to exclude serious spinal cord or cauda equina pathology.

- **Lower limb numbness/tingling/weakness**. These are 'hard' neurological symptoms and signs that demand urgent investigation to exclude spinal cord pathology.

- **Diurnal variation**. Simple mechanical back pain usually improves on rest and at night. Unremitting pain that keeps the patient awake is more likely to be due to malignancy or infection and is a 'red flag' sign (see **Hazard** on p. 274). Once again, urgent investigation is mandatory. Inflammatory back pain classically improves on exercise, is not relieved by rest and may wake the patient at night.

- **Stiffness**. One of the hallmarks of inflammatory arthritis is early morning stiffness that lasts for at least 30 minutes after rising.

- **Relationship to exercise**. The pain of inflammatory arthritis typically improves on exercise. Spinal stenosis, which is usually congenital, is often asymptomatic but may cause nerve root pain which starts after walking as the nerve roots swell and become compressed. The patient may complain of lower limb pain, numbness and buttock pain on walking.

- **Systemic symptoms**. The presence of weight loss, night sweats or fever also constitutes 'red flag' symptoms (see **Hazard** over the page), which require urgent investigation as they may indicate a malignant or infective aetiology.
  - Remember that tuberculosis (TB) is common in many countries in Africa, Asia and the Indian subcontinent, and that the likelihood of a diagnosis of TB is much higher in patients born in countries with a high incidence of TB, even if they have lived for many years in a low-incidence country.
  - Similarly, groups such as intravenous drug users have a much higher incidence of systemic staphylococcal infection. This can be responsible for localized discitis or osteomyelitis of the spine.

Referred pain

We listed some causes of back pain at the start of this chapter that originate in retroperitoneal structures such as the kidneys, pancreas and abdominal aorta. Generally, back pain from these sources will occur in addition to pain and symptoms at other sites, indicating that the spine is not the primary origin of the pain.

- Acute pyelonephritis usually causes loin pain and associated symptoms of urinary tract infection.
- Renal stones classically cause extreme colicky loin pain that radiates to the groin.
- Acute pancreatitis causes upper abdominal pain that may radiate to the back.
- A ruptured abdominal aortic aneurysm results in abdominal pain that may radiate to the back.
- Aortic dissection typically causes severe chest pain that radiates to the upper back and is described as 'tearing' in nature.

Some patients with these conditions present atypically and it is possible for back pain to be the primary presenting symptom of any of them.

THINK

How commonly is back pain caused by cancer?
Cancer accounts for less than 1 per cent of back pain presentations generally, but over 90 per cent of patients with a known history of cancer and new presentation of back pain have spine metastases.

HAZARD

Don't miss 'red flag' clinical features, all demanding urgent investigation. These include:

- back pain that is unremitting and keeps the patient awake at night
- the presence of abnormal neurological signs
- fever
- immunosuppression
- weight loss
- history of cancer
- duration longer than 6 weeks
- osteoporosis
- use of long-term corticosteroids
- age over 70.

HAZARD

Cauda equina syndrome is a medical emergency caused by a central lumbar disc protrusion below the L1 vertebra. The spinal cord finishes at L1 in most adults and, below this level, multiple nerve roots will be compressed by any centrally prolapsed disc or protruding tumour.

Clinical features of cauda equina syndrome include:
- urinary retention with overflow
- constipation
- saddle anaesthesia
- bilateral leg weakness
- symptoms and signs of nerve root compression.

● Examination

General examination

If any systemic or 'red flag' features are detected, a full general examination is mandatory looking in particular for evidence of malignancy or infection. Examine for the following.

- **Fever**. This is indicative of infection.
- **Lymphadenopathy**. This may be present in disseminated malignancy or infection.
- **Cachexia**. This is a feature of advanced malignancy.
- **Breast lumps**.
- **Lower limb weakness, numbness, increased tone or brisk reflexes**. These are possible indicators of spinal cord compression.
- **A sensory level**. This is defined as loss of sensation below a particular dermatome and is highly suggestive of spinal cord compression above that level.
- **Urinary retention**. This too is a symptom suggestive of spinal cord compression or of compression of the cauda equina.
- **Rectal examination**. Loss of anal tone too is a sign of compression of either the spinal cord or the cauda equina. In the latter case, there may well be associated loss of sensation in a 'saddle distribution' (see Chapter 11).
- **Prostate**. In men, examination of the prostate gland is important, to look for evidence of malignancy.

THINK

Which malignancies most commonly metastasize to bone?

Lung, breast, prostate, thyroid and renal malignancies.

Specific examination of the back

This should include the following.

- **Inspection for muscle spasm and scoliosis**.
- **Assessment of range of movement**.
- **Palpation for spinal tenderness**. This is common in osteoporotic fracture, infection and malignancy.
- **Straight leg raise**. This is tested with the patient supine to look for radiculopathy. This is considered to be present if the pain of sciatica can be reproduced by less than 60 degrees of passive elevation with the ankle in dorsiflexion.
- **Sciatica**. Evaluation of L5 and S1 nerve roots if sciatica is present:
  - L5 motor function can be tested by evaluating dorsiflexion of the foot and of the big toe.
  - L5 sensory function is represented by sensation of the medial foot and the web space between the first and second toes.
  - S1 motor function can be tested by evaluating ankle jerks and sensory function by testing sensation over the posterior calf.

CLINICAL TIP

Ankle jerk reflexes often diminish with age, but usually bilaterally. In older patients it is worth checking both ankle jerks carefully. Bilateral reduction or loss of reflexes is common, but unilateral loss of an ankle jerk is more likely to be significant.

● Investigations

Acute low back pain in an otherwise well patient with no 'red flag' features does not automatically require investigation as most episodes are self-limiting. In all other cases, initial investigations should be guided by the following.

X-ray studies

Plain spine x-rays

These should be at a level appropriate for the pain – lumbar, thoracic or cervical. Both anteroposterior and lateral views should be performed. In patients of reproductive age, the gonadal radiation dose can be significant, particularly if x-rays are repeated. Plain spine x-rays can help greatly in the diagnosis of the following.

- *Osteoporosis and osteoporotic vertebral crush fracture.* Often no further imaging will be required.
- *Malignancy including myeloma.* Vertebral body destruction by sclerotic or lytic lesions (bone destruction due to malignant deposits) can be seen.
- *Infection.* Bone destruction extending across a disc space to involve adjacent vertebral bodies is suggestive of an infective process.
- *Spondylolisthesis and spondyloarthropathy.* These can be clearly visualized on plain films. For example, ankyloses between vertebral bodies can be seen in conditions such as ankylosing spondylitis.

CLINICAL TIP

Note that plain spine x-rays have significant limitations. They cannot reveal intervertebral disc prolapse and cannot assess nerve root or spinal cord compression. In addition, any pathological process usually has to be well established before it becomes visible on a plain spine x-ray; early or small lesions are commonly undetectable.

Chest x-ray

This is indicated if you suspect a previously undiagnosed lung cancer with spinal metastases. Note that you cannot adequately assess the thoracic spine on a chest x-ray (CXR).

THINK

What is the gonadal radiation dose from two views of the lumbar spine?
It is equivalent to more than 350 CXRs.

Computerized tomography and magnetic resonance imaging

Both CT and MRI provide vastly superior information compared with plain x-ray studies, particularly in the imaging of:

- intervertebral discs
- the spinal cord and nerve roots
- spinal or epidural infection
- malignancy (Figs 19.1 and 19.2).

MRI is to be preferred as it provides better imaging of soft tissue structures and does not involve a radiation dose. The radiological investigation of choice, therefore, in assessing back pain with any 'red flag' features, is MRI. It allows detailed imaging of nerve roots and the spinal cord. Disc prolapse can also be clearly visualized.

Further invasive investigations can be guided by MRI and CT if material is needed from the affected area for histology or microbiology.

Radionuclide bone scanning

Commonly known as a 'bone scan', this test involves scanning the whole skeleton following injection of a radioactive isotope. The isotope is taken up by metabolically active tissue in bone

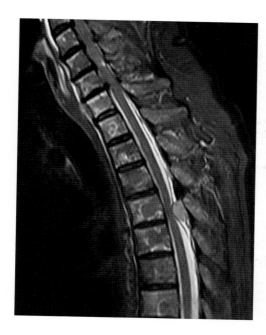

Fig. 19.1 Magnetic resonance imaging of a patient with diffuse spine metastases due to lung cancer. Note the multiple lesions of differing density in every vertebral body

and can indicate sites of metastases, infection and increased bone turnover such as may occur in healing fractures and active arthritis. Although useful as a 'screening' test for skeletal metastases and occult infection, the images are inferior to MRI for precise characterization. Further investigation is usually warranted with MRI if abnormalities are detected.

Blood and laboratory tests

If a serious aetiology for back pain is suspected then various blood tests might be indicated depending on the differential diagnosis.

Infective causes

- Full blood count, C-reactive protein, blood cultures, HIV test.
- *If tuberculosis is suspected*, a serum QuantiFERON® or a skin tuberculin (Mantoux) test may be helpful. However, be aware that a positive result in either case may be due to latent rather

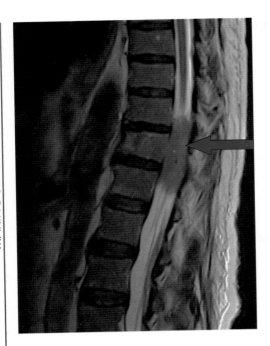

Fig. 19.2 Magnetic resonance imaging showing a metastasis at T11 with epidural extension (arrowed). This patient presented with symptoms of spinal cord compression at T11

than active TB. Conversely, a negative QuantiFERON® or Mantoux test does not exclude active TB. We recommend seeking specialist advice from a respiratory or infectious diseases physician *early* if a diagnosis of spinal TB is suspected.

Malignant causes including myeloma

- Full blood count, serum calcium, serum protein electrophoresis, tumour markers (e.g. prostate-specific antigen in men and CA15-3 for breast cancer in women).
- Examination of the urine for a monoclonal protein band (Bence Jones protein) is important in the investigation of potential multiple myeloma.

Inflammatory causes

- ESR and C-reactive protein as inflammatory markers.
- Rheumatoid factor for suspected rheumatoid arthritis.
- HLA B27 if ankylosing spondylitis is a possibility.

Making the diagnosis

A diagnosis is usually reached using a combination of the history, examination and investigations, particularly MRI where 'red flag' features are present. CT-guided aspiration of an area considered to be infective or malignant in nature may be needed to confirm a causative infective organism or tumour. In a patient with a prior diagnosis of cancer having a propensity to metastasize to bone, tissue confirmation may not be necessary if clear evidence of metastasis is seen on MRI – a specialist opinion will be required from an oncologist.

If investigations fail to provide a satisfactory explanation for the patient's back pain, then other potential diagnostic explanations must be considered and these include the possibility of pain referred from retroperitoneal structures as mentioned above.

20 Leg swelling

Introduction

The symptom of leg swelling encompasses a broad spectrum of diagnoses, ranging from a simple, localized problem such as venous stasis resulting from prolonged immobility to a symptom suggestive of serious cardiac, renal, hepatic or respiratory disease.

The most common causes of leg swelling in patients presenting to acute medical services are:

- *unilateral* – deep-vein thrombosis (DVT) and cellulitis
- *bilateral* – congestive cardiac failure and venous stasis from prolonged sitting.

There is a more detailed differential diagnosis, of course, and a practical classification of this is presented here.

● Classification of leg swelling

Oedematous swelling

Oedematous leg swelling is identified by the presence of pitting oedema. This is usually bilateral. The swelling starts in the legs and may ascend with increasing severity to include the abdominal wall or sacrum (particularly if the patient has been lying in bed). It may also result in ascites.

- Venous stasis:
  - Deep-vein thrombosis (DVT). The presentation will depend on the site of the thrombosis. A lower limb DVT may present with localized swelling of one calf only. A proximal DVT extending into the iliac veins or inferior vena cava will present with much more extensive and possibly bilateral swelling
  - Prolonged sitting with the legs down (common)
  - Pregnancy – because of pressure on the pelvic veins from the pregnant uterus (common)
  - Pelvic tumour obstructing venous return (uncommon)
- Congestive (biventricular) cardiac failure:
  - Ischaemic heart disease
  - Cardiomyopathy
  - Valvular heart disease
- Right ventricular failure due to pulmonary hypertension:
  - Primary (e.g. primary pulmonary hypertension – uncommon)
  - Secondary to advanced chronic lung disease such as chronic obstructive pulmonary disease (COPD), bronchiectasis or pulmonary fibrosis – this is known as cor pulmonale and is common
  - Other important but less common causes of secondary pulmonary hypertension include chronic

thromboembolic pulmonary hypertension, obesity hypoventilation syndrome, obstructive sleep apnoea, mitral stenosis, appetite-suppressant drugs such as dexfenfluramine, and HIV infection

- Hypoproteinaemic states:
  - Chronic liver failure
  - Nephrotic syndrome
  - Protein-losing enteropathy
  - Protein malnutrition (rare in developed countries)
- Primary renal disease (e.g. acute nephritic syndrome, which leads to salt and water retention and oedema)
- Drugs causing vasodilatation (commonly the calcium-channel blockers, particularly nifedipine)
- Constrictive pericarditis (rare in developed countries)

Non-oedematous leg swelling (non-pitting)

This is most often unilateral. The principal causes are as listed here.

- Cellulitis
- Lymphoedema (this usually presents as a long-standing problem of insidious onset caused by lymphatic obstruction. Limb swelling due to lymphoedema can be massive and the skin feels thickened and rough to the touch. The presence of lymphoedema predisposes the patient to episodes of cellulitis in the affected limb.)
  - Primary lymphoedema is congenital and is due to an inherited deficiency of lymphatic vessels (Milroy's syndrome).
  - Secondary lymphoedema can be caused by malignant obstruction of lymphatic drainage. Another cause in developing countries is filariasis, a parasitic infection where the presence of filarial worms is directly responsible for lymphatic obstruction.

What are the basic mechanisms of causation of oedema?

- Raised venous pressure is one, such as occurs in congestive cardiac failure (CCF), right ventricular failure or venous stasis.
- Salt retention can occur in primary renal disease such as nephritic syndrome, or can be secondary to the hyperaldosteronism induced by poor cardiac output or cirrhosis.
- Another mechanism is reduced intravascular oncotic pressure due to hypoproteinaemic states.

Note that some causes – cirrhosis and CCF are examples – cause oedema through more than one mechanism.

History

Salient points in the history that aid diagnosis include the following.

- **Speed of onset**. DVT or cellulitis usually develops over the course of a few days. Patients with CCF usually develop oedema over days or weeks. Some of the causes listed above have an insidious onset and so a much longer history; examples are the oedema associated with pulmonary hypertension, cirrhosis and lymphoedema.
- **Degree of mobility**. Is the patient normally freely mobile, or does he or she spend hours a day sitting in a chair with their legs down? Immobility increases the likelihood of dependent oedema by causing venous stasis.
- **Localized pain, redness and inflammation**. The presence of these symptoms increases the likelihood of cellulitis, particularly in a patient with diabetes. Ask about possible routes of infection such as recent insect bites and local skin trauma.

- **Medical history**. A history of CCF increases the likelihood of a recurrent episode of heart failure. Ask carefully about pre-existing cardiac, respiratory, liver and renal disease. Long-standing respiratory disease such as chronic obstructive pulmonary disease (COPD), bronchiectasis or pulmonary fibrosis may suggest cor pulmonale. A previous proven DVT also increases the risk of recurrent thromboembolism.

- **Drugs**. You may get clues as to possible aetiology from looking at the patient's drug history. A long list of drugs for cardiac disease increases the likelihood of CCF. Look in particular for calcium-channel blockers as these are a potent cause of oedema.

- **Associated symptoms**. Breathlessness and orthopnoea may suggest pulmonary oedema, increasing the likelihood of a diagnosis of CCF.

- **Alcohol intake**. An accurate alcohol history is vital in assessing the risk of chronic liver disease (see Chapter 15).

- **Risk factors for DVT**. The likelihood of a diagnosis of DVT rises significantly in the presence of risk factors for venous thromboembolism. Risk factors for pulmonary embolism are covered in detail in Chapter 3.

THINK

What are the risk factors for venous thromboembolism?
The major risk factors for VTE are:
- immobility
- active cancer
- recent lower limb surgery or fracture
- pregnancy
- previous VTE
- thrombophilia.

The oral contraceptive pill and long-haul air travel are relatively minor risk factors.

● Examination

Distribution

Is the swelling unilateral or bilateral? Unilateral swelling is more suggestive of cellulitis or DVT. Most of the other causes presenting in an acute medical setting will cause bilateral swelling.

Evidence of infection

If the swollen area is hot, inflamed and tender, then cellulitis is the likely diagnosis. Look in this case for a source of infection (see **Think** over the page) and consider a diagnosis of necrotizing fasciitis if the patient is systemically unwell (see **Hazard** over the page).

Pitting

Swelling is classically described as oedematous if it is 'pitting'. This is defined as an indentation that remains for some minutes after pressing on the swollen limb with fingertips. If pitting oedema is present, look for the following.

CCF

Signs are:

- tachycardia
- raised respiratory rate
- inspiratory crackles at the lung bases
- pleural effusions
- raised jugular venous pressure (JVP).

Underlying cardiac disease

Signs are:

- heart murmurs
- added heart sounds
- left ventricular or right ventricular enlargement or hypertrophy.

Chronic liver disease

Signs are:

- jaundice
- spider naevi
- palmar erythema
- leuconychia
- ascites
- bruising, poor nutrition and muscle wasting.

Cor pulmonale as a result of chronic respiratory disease

- JVP is usually elevated and the patient may be centrally cyanosed breathing room air, and tachypnoeic as well.
- Cor pulmonale occurs as a result of long-standing and advanced ('end stage') respiratory disease.
- Patients with advanced COPD are commonly wheezy and have hyperinflated lungs, with accessory muscle use and a barrel-chested appearance.
- Patients with pulmonary fibrosis will have bilateral inspiratory crackles that do not change on coughing and they may have finger clubbing.
- Patients with advanced bronchiectasis may have finger clubbing and will probably have extensive inspiratory and expiratory crackles that change on coughing because they are generated by the presence of sputum in the airways.

Nephrotic syndrome

As well as bilateral lower limb oedema, pleural effusions, oedema involving the face and arms, sometimes ascites may also be present. Heavy proteinuria will be apparent.

THINK

What sources of infection should be considered in a patient with lower limb cellulitis?
Look for cuts and breaks in the skin around the feet and lower legs. Look in particular for evidence of *Tinea pedis* ('athlete's foot') with cracks between the toes.

This is very common in association with cellulitis and it requires aggressive treatment with topical and oral antifungal agents.

⚡ HAZARD

In a patient with rapidly progressing cellulitis or signs of systemic sepsis with cellulitis, a diagnosis of necrotizing fasciitis should be considered. This condition is classified into type 1 (mainly affecting diabetic patients and caused by a combination of aerobic and anaerobic bacteria) and type 2 (which can affect previously healthy subjects and is caused by group A streptococci). Necrotizing fasciitis is a medical emergency with a high mortality and it demands immediate intravenous antibiotics and surgical debridement.

● Investigations

General

Most causes of leg swelling can be confidently diagnosed with a competent history and examination, supplemented by a few, relatively simple, tests available in an emergency department or acute medical admitting unit. The exact combination of tests should be tailored to the suspected diagnosis. For example, if you strongly suspect a DVT or cellulitis then not all of the blood or radiological tests listed below will be required.

- *Full blood count.* Look for a raised white cell count and neutrophilia if you suspect cellulitis.
- *Urea and electrolytes.* Look for renal impairment in an oedematous patient. If present it may indicate primary renal disease (such as nephritic syndrome), and in patients with other causes of oedema (such as CCF and chronic liver disease) it will impact on your management with drugs

such as diuretics. In either case, careful subsequent monitoring of renal function is mandatory.

- *Liver function tests.* A serum albumin of <30 g/L may indicate a hypoproteinaemic state. Other liver enzymes may be deranged in chronic liver disease. For a more comprehensive discussion, see Chapter 15.
- *C-reactive protein.* This is likely to be elevated in cellulitis.
- *D-dimer.* Use this test selectively. It is often used indiscriminately as a screening test for venous thromboembolism and this is inappropriate.
  - If the D-dimer is negative in a low-risk patient then it has high negative predictive value for DVT and the diagnosis can be confidently ruled out.
  - If, on the other hand, the patient has one or more risk factors for venous thromboembolism, a negative result is less reliable and further investigation is required to exclude a DVT.
  - A positive result can arise in many clinical circumstances and is not diagnostic of DVT.

THINK

What are the causes of a positive D-dimer other than venous thromboembolism?

Causes are: infection; immobility; malignancy; pregnancy; recent surgery. Most hospital inpatients will have a raised D-dimer after a couple of days in hospital.

- *Brain natriuretic peptide* (BNP). This is a protein released by myocardial cells. Its name refers to the fact that it was first identified in the brain.
  - Levels of BNP rise in cardiac failure. The advent of quick and reliable BNP assays will probably lead to the routine use of this test in the future.
  - A normal level in a breathless patient makes cardiac failure very unlikely.

- BNP is excreted by the kidney, so caution must be exercised in interpreting results in patients with renal failure.
- *Urine dipstick for protein.* This is a quick and easy screen for proteinuria. If persistently positive in the context of oedema with + + + or more then nephritic syndrome or nephrotic syndrome may be possible diagnoses. A quantification of daily total protein excretion will be indicated. This has traditionally been performed by means of a 24 hour urine collection but patients often find this onerous and the results can be unreliable. An easier and quicker method is to send an early morning urine sample for measurement of the protein creatinine ratio (PCR). 'Nephrotic range' proteinuria is a PCR of >350 mg/mmol which equates to a daily protein excretion of greater than about 3.5 g. If the serum albumin is below 30 g/L in an oedematous patient with a PCR in the nephrotic range then nephrotic syndrome is likely. A normal PCR is defined as <15 mg/mmol and levels above this (but below the nephrotic range) in the context of oedema and renal impairment may indicate primary renal disease such as nephritic syndrome. Specialist renal referral will be indicated in this situation.
- *Electrocardiogram.* This is almost always abnormal in CCF, so a normal ECG should prompt consideration of an alternative reason for oedema.
    - Common abnormalities in CCF include atrial fibrillation, multiple ventricular ectopic beats or bigeminy, left bundle branch block, first-degree heart block, evidence of ischaemia or previous infarction.
    - In cor pulmonale and other causes of pulmonary hypertension, the ECG may show tall P waves (above about 2.5 mm in height) in leads II, III and aVF. This appearance is referred to as P pulmonale and it is due to right atrial enlargement. There may also be evidence of right ventricular hypertrophy with right axis deviation and a dominant R wave in V1.

- Chest x-ray
  - This will confirm a diagnosis of CCF in most cases. Look for cardiac enlargement, small bilateral pleural effusions, peripheral septal lines (often referred to as 'Kerley B' lines in other texts) and upper lobe venous distension. These are all radiographic features of pulmonary oedema and pulmonary venous congestion.
  - If you suspect cor pulmonale, look for evidence of chronic lung disease such as COPD (lung hyperinflation, bullae), pulmonary fibrosis (reticulonodular shadowing) or bronchiectasis (tramline and ring shadows).
- *Doppler ultrasound of deep leg veins*. This is the investigation of choice to confirm a diagnosis of DVT.

Further investigations

Once you have ascertained the likely cause of leg swelling, then further investigations may be needed.

- *Echocardiogram*. If a diagnosis of CCF or right ventricular failure is confirmed with initial investigations, an echocardiogram is indicated in order to determine the degree and type of cardiac impairment. Valvular heart disease or cardiomyopathy may also be identified and referral to a cardiologist may be indicated. Pulmonary hypertension can be confirmed by echocardiography.
- *Lung function tests*. These will be indicated if you suspect cor pulmonale or pulmonary hypertension from any cause. The pattern of abnormality may point to possible causes of chronic lung disease. For instance, a severe obstructive defect can confirm a clinical diagnosis of COPD and a restrictive defect can confirm a clinical diagnosis of pulmonary fibrosis. In many cases of pulmonary hypertension, lung function testing does not provide a clear diagnosis, however. The results will need to be interpreted by an expert and other investigations such as chest CT scanning are likely to be required. A diagnosis of pulmonary hypertension from any cause

is an indication for a prompt referral to a respiratory physician.

- *Liver ultrasound*. This is indicated if chronic liver disease is suspected. Referral to a hepatologist will also be indicated.
- *Renal tract ultrasound*. Further investigation of the renal tract is indicated in suspected nephrotic syndrome or when renal impairment is present. Referral to a renal physician will be indicated.
  - Renal tract obstruction (possible causes are renal calculi, retroperitoneal fibrosis or prostatic hypertrophy) will be quickly identified.
  - The size of the kidneys is also helpful. Normal sized kidneys in the context of renal impairment indicate a fairly acute cause such as acute nephritis; whereas small, scarred kidneys suggest a chronic problem, such as hypertensive nephropathy.

Index